T0212979

Lecture Notes in Computer Science   10550

Commenced Publication in 1973
Founding and Former Series Editors:
Gerhard Goos, Juris Hartmanis, and Jan van Leeuwen

More information about this series at http://www.springer.com/series/7412

M. Jorge Cardoso · Tal Arbel et al. (Eds.)

Computer Assisted and Robotic Endoscopy and Clinical Image-Based Procedures

4th International Workshop, CARE 2017
and 6th International Workshop, CLIP 2017
Held in Conjunction with MICCAI 2017
Québec City, QC, Canada, September 14, 2017
Proceedings

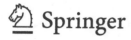

Springer

Editors
M. Jorge Cardoso
University College London
London
UK

Tal Arbel
McGill University
Montreal, QC
Canada

Workshop Editors *see next page*

ISSN 0302-9743 ISSN 1611-3349 (electronic)
Lecture Notes in Computer Science
ISBN 978-3-319-67542-8 ISBN 978-3-319-67543-5 (eBook)
DOI 10.1007/978-3-319-67543-5

Library of Congress Control Number: 2017953402

LNCS Sublibrary: SL6 – Image Processing, Computer Vision, Pattern Recognition, and Graphics

Printed on acid-free paper

This Springer imprint is published by Springer Nature
The registered company is Springer International Publishing AG
The registered company address is: Gewerbestrasse 11, 6330 Cham, Switzerland

Workshop Editors

4th International Workshop on Computer Assisted and Robotic Endoscopy, CARE 2017

Jonathan McLeod
University of Western Ontario
London, ON
Canada

Terry Peters
University of Western Ontario
London, ON
Canada

Tobias Reichl
KUKA Laboratories GmbH
Augsburg
Germany

Kensaku Mori
Nagoya University
Nagoya
Japan

Xiongbiao Luo
Xiamen University
Xiamen
China

Andreas Uhl
University of Salzburg
Salzburg
Austria

6th International Workshop on Clinical Image-Based Procedures, CLIP 2017

Klaus Drechsler
Fraunhofer IGD
Darmstadt
Germany

Cristina Oyarzun Laura
Fraunhofer IGD
Darmstadt
Germany

Marius Erdt
Fraunhofer Singapore
Singapore
Singapore

Raj Shekhar
Children's National Health System
Washington, DC
USA

Miguel Ángel González Ballester
ICREA – Universitat Pompeu Fabra
Barcelona
Spain

Stefan Wesarg
Fraunhofer IGD
Darmstadt
Germany

Marius George Linguraru
Children's National Health System
Washington, DC
USA

Preface CARE 2017

The 4th International Workshop on Computer-Assisted Robotic Endoscopy (CARE 2017) was held in conjunction with MICCAI on September 14th, 2017 in Quebec City, Canada. Building on the success of the previous three workshops, CARE 2017 brought together researchers, clinicians, and medical companies to advance the field of computer-assisted and robotic endoscopy.

This workshop featured high-quality original papers and invited keynote presentations on the latest advances in computer-assisted and robotic endoscopy. After peer review, seven papers were selected for presentation at CARE 2017 and are included in these proceedings. As in previous years, CARE 2017 included keynote presentations from leading experts in academia and industry. This year we were honoured to have Dr. Dan Stoyanov (University College London, UK) and Dr. Michael Wood (Synaptive Medical, Canada) give keynote presentations for the workshop.

We would like to thank all the reviewers and members of the programme committee who contributed their time, effort and expertise to make this workshop possible. We are grateful to all the authors and attendees for their scientific research and enthusiastic participation in CARE 2017. We would also like to express our gratitude to the organizers of MICCAI for supporting this workshop and to KUKA Robotics for sponsoring the best paper awards.

September 2017

Jonathan McLeod
Tobias Reichl
Xiongbiao Luo
Terry Peters
Kensaku Mori
Andreas Uhl

Organization

Organizing Committee

Jonathan McLeod — Western University, Canada
Tobias Reichl — KUKA Laboratories GmbH, Germany
Xiongbiao Luo — Xiamen University, China
Terry Peters — Western University, Canada
Kensaku Mori — Nagoya University, Japan
Andreas Uhl — University of Salzburg, Austria

Program Committee

John S.H. Baxter — Western University, Canada
Toby Collins — Université d'Auvergne, France
Nishikant Deshmukh — Johns Hopkins University, USA
Luis Garcia-Peraza Herrera — University College London, UK
Stamatia Giannarou — Imperial College London, UK
Uditha Jarayathne — Western University, Canada
Nader Mahmoud — Université de Strasbourg, France
Peter Mountney — Siemens Healthcare
Krittin Pachtrachai — University College London, UK
Austin Reiter — Johns Hopkins University, USA
Nima Tajbakhsh — Arizona State University, USA
Andreas Uhl — University of Salzburg, Austria
Wenyao Xia — Western University, Canada
Menglong Ye — Imperial College London, UK

Preface CLIP 2017

On September 14, 2017, the 6th International Workshop on Clinical Image-Based Procedures: From Planning to Intervention (CLIP 2017) was held in Quebec City, Quebec, Canada in conjunction with the 20th International Conference on Medical Image Computing and Computer Assisted Intervention (MICCAI). Following the tradition set in the last five years, this year's workshop was an exciting forum for the discussion and dissemination of clinically tested, state-of-the-art methods for image-based planning, monitoring, and evaluation of medical procedures, as in previous years.

Over the past few years, there has been considerable and growing interest in the development and evaluation of new translational image-based techniques in the modern hospital. For a decade or more, a proliferation of meetings dedicated to medical image computing has created a need for greater study and scrutiny of the clinical application and validation of such methods. New attention and new strategies are essential to ensure a smooth and effective translation of computational image-based techniques into the clinic. For these reasons and to complement other technology-focused MICCAI workshops on computer-assisted interventions, CLIP 2017's major focus continued to be on filling the gaps between basic science and clinical applications.

Members of the medical imaging community were encouraged to submit work centered on specific clinical applications, including techniques and procedures based on clinical data or already in use and evaluated by clinical users. Once again, the event brought together world-class researchers and clinicians who presented ways to strengthen links between computer scientists and engineers, and surgeons, interventional radiologists, and radiation oncologists.

In response to the call for papers, 12 original manuscripts were submitted for presentation at CLIP 2017. Each of the manuscripts underwent a meticulous double-blind peer review by three members of the Program Committee, all of them prestigious experts in the field of medical image analysis and clinical translations of technology. A member of the Organizing Committee further oversaw the review of each manuscript. Ten manuscripts were accepted for oral presentation at the workshop. The accepted contributors represented nine countries from three continents: Europe, North America, and Asia. Judging by the contributions received, the quality of CLIP 2017 improved compared with last year's event. However, we also noticed that the number of submissions decreased compared with the events of the last two years. This might be due to the increasing number of satellite events around the MICCAI main conference.

As always, the workshop featured a prominent expert as keynoter. Underscoring the translational, bench-to-bedside theme of the workshop, the CLIP 2017 keynote was given by Neil Glossop, a recognized expert in the field of image-guided surgery from ArciTrax Inc. and the University of Toronto.

We would like to acknowledge the invaluable contribution of our entire Program Committee, many members of which have actively participated in the planning of the workshop over the years, and without whose assistance CLIP 2017 would not have been possible. Our thanks also go to all the authors in this volume for the high quality of their work and their commitment of time and effort. Finally, we are grateful to the MICCAI organizers for supporting the organization of CLIP 2017.

September 2017   Stefan Wesarg
Miguel Ángel González Ballester
Klaus Drechsler
Marius Erdt
Marius George Linguraru
Cristina Oyarzun Laura
Raj Shekhar

Organization

Organizing Committee

Klaus Drechsler	Fraunhofer IGD, Germany
Marius Erdt	Fraunhofer, Singapore
Miguel Ángel González Ballester	Universitat Pompeu Fabra, Spain
Marius George Linguraru	Children's National Health System, USA
Cristina Oyarzun Laura	Fraunhofer IGD, Germany
Raj Shekhar	Children's National Health System, USA
Stefan Wesarg	Fraunhofer IGD, Germany

Program Committee

Juan Cerrolaza	Imperial College, UK
Yufei Chen	Tongji University, China
Jan Egger	TU Graz, Austria
Moti Freiman	Philips Healthcare, Israel
Tobias Heimann	Siemens Healthcare GmbH, Germany
Xin Kang	Sonavex Inc., USA
Yogesh Karpate	Children's National Medical Center, USA
Jianfei Liu	National Institutes of Health, USA
Xinyang Liu	Children's National Health System, USA
Awais Mansoor	Children's National Medical Center, USA
Antonio R. Porras	Children's National Health System, USA
Carles Sanchez	Computer Vision Center (UAB), Spain
Jiayin Zhou	Institute for Infocomm Research, Singapore
Stephan Zidowitz	Fraunhofer MEVIS, Germany

Contents

4th International Workshop on Computer Assisted and Robotic Endoscopy, CARE 2017

Shape-Based Pose Estimation of Robotic Surgical Instruments 3
 Daniel Wesierski and Sebastian Cygert

3D Endoscope System Using Asynchronously Blinking Grid Pattern
Projection for HDR Image Synthesis 16
 *Ryo Furukawa, Masahito Naito, Daisuke Miyazaki, Masahi Baba,
 Shinsaku Hiura, Yoji Sanomura, Shinji Tanaka,
 and Hiroshi Kawasaki*

Towards Real-Time Polyp Detection in Colonoscopy Videos: Adapting
Still Frame-Based Methodologies for Video Sequences Analysis 29
 *Quentin Angermann, Jorge Bernal, Cristina Sánchez-Montes,
 Maroua Hammami, Gloria Fernández-Esparrach, Xavier Dray,
 Olivier Romain, F. Javier Sánchez, and Aymeric Histace*

Progressive Hand-Eye Calibration for Laparoscopic Surgery Navigation 42
 *Jinliang Shao, Huoling Luo, Deqiang Xiao, Qingmao Hu,
 and Fucang Jia*

Learning Camera Pose from Optical Colonoscopy Frames Through Deep
Convolutional Neural Network (CNN) 50
 *Mohammad Ali Armin, Nick Barnes, Jose Alvarez, Hongdong Li,
 Florian Grimpen, and Olivier Salvado*

Motion Vector for Outlier Elimination in Feature Matching
and Its Application in SLAM Based Laparoscopic Tracking 60
 *Cheng Wang, Masahiro Oda, Yuichiro Hayashi, Kazunari Misawa,
 Holger Roth, and Kensaku Mori*

Image-Based Smoke Detection in Laparoscopic Videos 70
 *Andreas Leibetseder, Manfred Jürgen Primus, Stefan Petscharnig,
 and Klaus Schoeffmann*

6th International Workshop on Clinical Image-Based Procedures, CLIP 2017

Fully Automatic Detection of Distal Radius Fractures from Posteroanterior
and Lateral Radiographs 91
 Raja Ebsim, Jawad Naqvi, and Tim Cootes

Automated Characterization of Pyelocalyceal Anatomy Using CT
Urograms to Aid in Management of Kidney Stones.................   99
   Yuankai Huo, Vaughn Braxton, S. Duke Herrell, Bennett Landman,
   and Smita De

Local Phase-Based Learning for Needle Detection and Localization
in 3D Ultrasound   108
   Cosmas Mwikirize, John L. Nosher, and Ilker Hacihaliloglu

Intracranial Volume Quantification from 3D Photography   116
   Liyun Tu, Antonio R. Porras, Scott Ensel, Deki Tsering,
   Beatriz Paniagua, Andinet Enquobahrie, Albert Oh,
   Robert Keating, Gary F. Rogers, and Marius George Linguraru

Automatic Near Real-Time Evaluation of 3D Ultrasound Scan Adequacy
for Developmental Dysplasia of the Hip.......................   124
   Olivia Paserin, Kishore Mulpuri, Anthony Cooper, Antony J. Hodgson,
   and Rafeef Abugharbieh

Automatic Sentinel Lymph Node Localization in Head and Neck
Cancer Using a Coupled Shape Model Algorithm...................   133
   Florian Jung, Biebl-Rydlo Medea, Jean-François Daisne,
   and Stefan Wesarg

Towards an Automated Segmentation of the Ventro-Intermediate
Thalamic Nucleus.....................................   141
   Elena Najdenovska, Constantin Tuleasca, João Jorge,
   José P. Marques, Philippe Maeder, Jean-Philippe Thiran,
   Marc Levivier, and Meritxell Bach Cuadra

Classification of Confocal Endomicroscopy Patterns for Diagnosis
of Lung Cancer......................................   151
   Debora Gil, Oriol Ramos-Terrades, Elisa Minchole, Carles Sanchez,
   Noelia Cubero de Frutos, Marta Diez-Ferrer, Rosa Maria Ortiz,
   and Antoni Rosell

Automated Classification for Breast Cancer Histopathology Images:
Is Stain Normalization Important?..........................   160
   Vibha Gupta, Apurva Singh, Kartikeya Sharma, and Arnav Bhavsar

Hybrid Tracking for Improved Registration of Laparoscopic Ultrasound
and Laparoscopic Video for Augmented Reality   170
   William Plishker, Xinyang Liu, and Raj Shekhar

Author Index   181

4th International Workshop on Computer Assisted and Robotic Endoscopy, CARE 2017

Shape-Based Pose Estimation of Robotic Surgical Instruments

Daniel Wesierski[1,2]([✉]) and Sebastian Cygert[1]

[1] Multimedia Systems Department, Faculty of Electronics,
Telecommunications, and Informatics, Gdansk University of Technology,
Gdansk, Poland
daniel.wesierski@pg.edu.pl
[2] Systems Research Institute, Polish Academy of Sciences,
Warsaw, Poland

Abstract. We describe a detector of robotic instrument parts in image-guided surgery. The detector consists of a huge ensemble of scale-variant and pose-dedicated, rigid appearance templates. The templates, which are equipped with pose-related keypoints and segmentation masks, allow for explicit pose estimation and segmentation of multiple end-effectors as well as fine-grained non-maximum suppression. We train the templates by grouping examples of end-effector articulations, imaged at various viewpoints, in thus arising space of instrument shapes. Proposed shape-based grouping forms tight clusters of pose-specific end-effector appearance. Experimental results show that the proposed method can effectively estimate the end-effector pose and delineate its boundary while being trained with moderately sized data clusters. We then show that matching such huge ensemble of templates takes less than one second on commodity hardware.

Keywords: Surgical instruments · Localization · Segmentation · Grouping

1 Introduction

Surgical robots with increased autonomy are an engaging objective for next-generation computer-aided intervention. A mature technology, though, very likely requires delivering visual algorithms that will grant robots full awareness of the operated surrounding. Precise and continuous localization of surgical instrument parts in images will then belong to primary robot abilities.

Scarcity of relevant data is one of the hurdles for traditional, data-driven approaches to tool part localization. Despite that the articulation of robotic instruments is not as free as, say, that of a human body, the available video snippets of specific surgeries usually contain only several tool motions. Efforts to account for incomplete spectrum of object articulations in available datasets usually consist in developing algorithms that should generalize to previously unseen object configurations. Alternatively, memory-centric methods only improve with

M.J. Cardoso et al. (Eds.): CARE/CLIP 2017, LNCS 10550, pp. 3–15, 2017.
DOI: 10.1007/978-3-319-67543-5_1

growing volumes of data. Intuitively, data-driven algorithms with generalization capability should require less data than memory-centric methods. On the other hand, a *proof of generalization* to unseen pose types may require such data-driven algorithms to correctly and repeatedly predict tool articulations for all possible tool-camera configurations, for instance, up to quantization, before being commissioned into operating rooms – an evaluation procedure that would as well exhaustively test the efficacy of memory-centric methods.

This work embraces a memory-centric approach that explicitly learns a wide spectrum of instrument poses by leveraging shapes of segmented instruments. We propose to explain the articulated motion of robotic surgical instruments with an ensemble of *scale-variant* and *pose-dedicated* appearance models. Learning the appearance of surgical instruments at different poses is challenged by image noise that appears, for instance, as blurry tool surface with incident specular reflections. Arguably, the more training examples a procedure uses for training an appearance model, the less the noisy observations contaminate the model. Our contribution is twofold. Despite data scarcity, we show that our approach can be accurate in estimating end-effector pose using a modest number of examples per pose type. Then, we demonstrate that grouping the examples based on their segmented shapes produces tight appearance clusters of training examples. The clusters in turn allow learning effective end-effector models in the form of the huge ensemble of scale-variant and pose-dedicated templates that can be fast evaluated in the image.

2   Related Work

Image-based pose estimation of robotic surgical instruments has been substantially studied in the literature [3]. Successfully evaluated algorithms for locating robotic tools in videos would immediately find applications in computer-aided intervention. The algorithms could assess and help improve skills of novice surgeons during surgical training [13], provide experienced surgeons with force feedback [1] and other helpful and unobtrusive metadata [12], and in further stages of maturity enable robots to take over some surgical tasks from the surgeon during a surgery [17].

One of the main approaches to locating tools in images relies on brute-force search for a monolithic template that best matches the image evidence. When the template encodes object pose, top-down template matching is an attractive approach to pose estimation. Despite being commonly referred to as a naive approach to object detection, data-driven template matching requires training a template-based detector. Notably, given abridged training datasets and adverse occlusions at test-time, such as self-occlusions, occlusions by other objects, and truncation at image border, a procedure for training a precise and robust, template-based tool pose estimator is challenging.

A large ensemble of rotation-variant and scale-variant templates exhaustively searched for rigid surgical tools over all image locations in [2]. The proposed pipeline converted an entry image to semantic maps of scores and labels using an Adaboost classifier in the first stage. In the second stage, rotated and scaled versions of the SVM-trained templates aggregated either real-valued semantic scores or discrete semantic labels for final output of multiple rigid instruments. The spatial extent of the templates was regularized during SVM training by enforcing 4-connected pixels to have close values in order to account for irregular response maps of the first stage of the pipeline. Authors reported, however, that the smoothed templates produced no improvement in the performance of the tool detector. Implemented on GPU, the detector ran nearly in real-time and estimated location and orientation of a rigid suction tube in complex surgical image scenes.

Local feature-based methods attempt to estimate tool pose from a video in a bottom-up manner. Robotic da Vinci tools possess inherent features that were captured with region covariance descriptors in [11]. Multi-class, randomized trees classifier scored the feature descriptors. Extended Kalman filter fused thus obtained heatmaps of characteristic landmarks with a CAD tool model and robot kinematics to recover the pose of robotic tools in 3D, though without end-effector articulation. An approach that, in turn, entirely relied on image features was proposed in [15] to estimate 2D tool pose. Haar-like features, which represented multiple tool landmarks in an initial batch of video frames, were fed into a multiclass classifier. Scanning the classifier over an image pyramid at test-time produced a response map of score clouds that assessed hypothesized locations and scales of tool parts. Ransac algorithm fit a line to the cloud that estimated the orientation of the tool shaft. Then, weighted averaging of the clouds output the tool center of a rigid instrument. Orientation and center location of the instrument was jointly estimated in [16] utilizing a structured model of mixtures of tool parts. Dynamic programming matched a diverse set of pose-dedicated appearance templates that corresponded to end-effector and shaft parts. Selecting best shaft subparts along hypothesized shaft orientations during inference coped with varying shaft length, subject to truncation at the image border.

Segmentation can improve object detection by feeding classifiers solely with foreground features [7]. Moreover, characteristic object contours often suffice as visual cues for template-based object detection in cluttered scenes [5]. Then, a deep residual network in [6], that was trained for joint segmentation and localization of shaft and end-effector parts of non-rigid and robotic tools, outperformed the network that was trained to do either segmentation or localization alone. Optic flow and color images jointly fed a CNN to obtain tool region proposals in [13]. Relying solely on images, the algorithm retrieved the 2D center of robotic tools in challenging phantom data.

Auxiliary information, such as robot encoder readings, can be exploited to improve computational efficiency of the algorithms and tool pose estimation. Contracting curve density algorithm tracked shaft contours in [14]. Initialized with image-projected robot CAD model, the algorithm learned online color statistics of inner and outer image regions to separate the shaft from the background. However, the method included no end-effector features and the estimated mask of the shaft was sliding along the shaft. A Gaussian mixture model captured the distribution of color and texture features of robotic tool parts in [10]. The proposed probabilistic regime required class-specific manual segmentation of the tool parts in the initial frames. The conducted experiments showed that the algorithm segmented well the shaft and end-effector parts but struggled with finer classification of the end-effector into robotic head and forceps. Random forests classified the shaft, end-effector, and background [1] using color features that were manually segmented from the first video frame. At each time instant, the algorithm projected the model contours of robot parts onto the labeled image and aligned them with the contours of both segments under level-set framework. Additionally, optical flow supported the estimation of tool trajectory in the presence of fast motion of the tools. The pose was estimated in 3D but without specifying the locations of the forcep tips. In a follow up work in [4], a 2D tracker was developed using Hough voting and SIFT features to automatically initialize the 3D tracker of [1]. It required the known 3D tool pose for initialization that was available from the projection of the tool onto the image using robot kinematics.

Full 3D pose of robotic tools, *i.e.* together with the end-effector articulation, was estimated in real-time in [18]. The method first split the robot gripper into local parts, anchored at multiple, manually chosen keypoints. For efficiency and robustness to occlusions, the appearance of a subset of parts was learned in an online manner by generating only part examples that were consistent with the currently estimated tool pose in 3D. The LINE algorithm [5] enhanced image contours and efficiently matched rendered templates of part contours to the image. Prosac algorithm then verified score aggregations through their geometric consistency with respect to rendered part configurations over a polar grid. Lifting the 2D tool pose to 3D was realized with Extended Kalman filter and robot kinematics. Noting that surgeons often prefer to work in close proximity to tissue in [12], only 3D pose of the end-effector was estimated. Likewise, the LINE algorithm was employed to efficiently match a huge set of pose-specific templates that were rendered online from the fine-grained CAD model of the end-effector.

Our method relies solely on image cues and uses region descriptors to represent characteristic tool features. It segments end-effector parts and recovers 2D end-effector articulation in a top-down manner, in the spirit of metadata-transfer of exemplar-SVMs [8]. By training pose-specific templates, it differs from [8] by (i) grouping the training examples based on their segmentation masks instead of training an SVM for each single example and (ii) transferring metadata of pose along with segmentation mask at test time that are averaged over respective groups of examples. Although it uses no auxiliary information, such as robot encoder readings, processing our large set of templates for segmentation and pose estimation could be aided by such prior knowledge in a similar manner to approaches that rely on robot kinematics.

3   Shape-Based Pose Estimation

Shape deformations of a robotic end-effector result from its articulating parts and camera-instrument viewpoint changes. In this section, we describe a simple, top-down method for locating end-effector parts in images. We capture the varying appearance of the end-effector with an ensemble of monolithic templates. Each template is assigned with a dedicated pose skeleton and a canonical segmentation mask. The method employs a brute-force search for templates that best match the image evidence. Selected, top-performing templates then explicitly transfer the assigned metadata for segmenting and estimating the pose of the end-effector.

As the huge collection of templates encode many shape variations, top-down template matching is an attractive approach to object pose estimation. Despite being commonly referred to as naive, data-driven template matching requires training a template-based detector. Arguably, the more training examples a procedure uses for training an appearance model, the less the noisy observations contaminate the modeled templates. Grouping image examples thus allows filtering out noise from the training samples during learning, thereby emphasizing discriminative features of the tool appearance. At the same time, though, imprecise grouping might attenuate good features leading to poor performance of the trained model. While grouping the examples can be approached by leveraging annotated keypoints, manual annotations require additional supervision. In this work, we describe a procedure that produces tight appearance clusters of the training examples by leveraging their shape cues. As the shape masks may be obtained from an external segmentation module, shape-based grouping is thus an attractive approach to reducing the amount of supervision during learning appearance models. The flowchart of our method is depicted in Fig. 1.

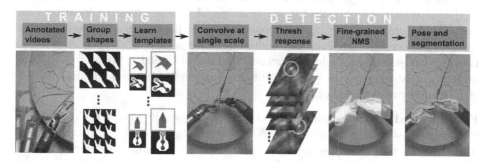

Fig. 1. Flowchart of our method. Given training video sequences of surgical instruments, we annotate pose-related keypoints and segmentation masks of the robotic end-effector. Proposed algorithm then uses (i) the segmentation masks for grouping and learning pose-dedicated appearance templates at training time and (ii) the skeleton keypoints for estimating the articulation of end-effectors at test-time. After convolving an entry image only at its original scale with the learned, huge set of pose-variant and scale-variant appearance templates, the selected templates, which best explain the image evidence after fine-grained non-maximum suppression (NMS), explicitly transfer the masks and the keypoints on the image, thereby estimating the pose as well as the shape of multiple robotic end-effectors.

3.1 Detection

Our method relies on brute-force search for the best template out of the huge set of templates at each image location. The templates encode tool appearance at various scales. Hence, they are convolved with an entry image only at single scale, without requiring to rescale the image in the pyramid-based manner.

Let I denote a two-dimensional image and $l \in \mathbb{N}^{2 \times 1}$ denote discrete locations in the image domain. The t-th template of the end-effector is denoted by w^t. It is associated with a segmentation mask m^t and a pose-specific keypoints k^t, thereby forming a 3-tuple $\{w^t, m^t, k^t\}_{t=1}^T$, where T is the total number of templates. Then, instantiating the templates in image I is scored as:

$$S(I, l, t) = w^t \phi^t(I, l) + b^t \tag{1}$$

where $\phi^t(I, l)$ is an image descriptor (e.g., histogram of oriented gradients, color histogram). The function $\phi^t(I, l)$ describes image region in the window of the t-th template at location l. The last term b^t is the bias, associated with the template, that relates to the size of the corresponding t-th cluster of examples.

Finding the template $\hat{t}$ at location $\hat{l}$ that best explains the whole image I is realized in a scanning window manner by solving:

$$(\hat{l}, \hat{t}) = \operatorname{argmax} S(I, l, t) \tag{2}$$

as depicted in the right part of Fig. 1. In effect, pose and segmentation mask of the detected $\hat{t}$-th end-effector are transferred to the image at location $\hat{l}$ as $\{m^{\hat{t}}, k^{\hat{t}}\}$. In practice, an image may contain more than one tool though. In this case, the procedure retrieves the highest scoring template at each each location $\hat{t}(l)$ and then thresholds the scores. Having obtained a table of candidate matches, it is necessary to suppress the non-maximal scoring candidates if they significantly overlap each other.

Fine-grained NMS. Non-maximum suppression greedily prunes the candidates that overlap with the top scoring candidate, selected at each iteration. Having direct access to the segmentation masks m^t of the candidate detections and to their precomputed areas, the algorithm can efficiently evaluate fine-grained extent of the overlap between an instantiated pair of candidates, for instance, of two end-effectors performing some grasping task close to each other (Fig. 1). The procedure is iteratively repeated until no candidates are left in the table.

3.2 Learning

We learn the parameters of the template ensemble in a supervised manner. The template models are learned separately and have the form $\beta^t = [b^t, w^t]$. The linear function (1) can be factored as $S(I_n, l, t) = \beta x_n$, where $x_n = (1, \phi^t(I_n, l))$ is a training feature vector for the t-th template.

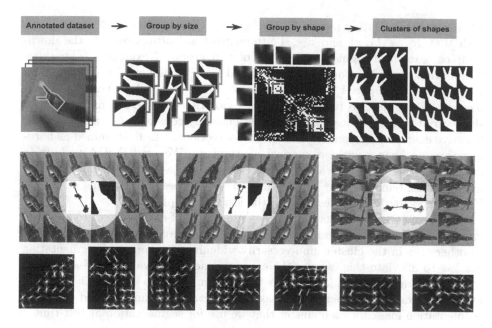

Fig. 2. Shape-based grouping of training examples from an annotated dataset.

Grouping. Assigning the example to respective t-th cluster, given its segmentation mask, is illustrated in Fig. 2. The algorithm proceeds in three steps. First, training examples are grouped by the sizes of their bounding boxes. The rectangular boxes are cropped to the extent of the segmentation masks of the examples. Second, each group of equally sized bounding boxes is split into subgroups that contain similar segmentation masks. The similarity of the segmentation masks is measured using the distance transform of pairs of examples. After thresholding the similarity scores, the procedure obtains a symmetric, binary co-occurrence table, that maps examples to clusters. Notably, the clusters can overlap each other. Finally, the obtained groups of pose-variant and scale-variant masks translate to groups of example clusters. Each cluster contains pose-specific keypoints and canonical segmentation mask, here encircled in the cluster centers. The keypoints are means of point clouds while the canonical mask results from binary sum of the masks of the clustered training examples.

Having grouped the examples, we learn regularized parameters of each template model β^t in a linear, asymmetric-cost SVM setting:

$$\text{argmin}_{\beta^t,\xi} \quad \frac{1}{2}\|\beta^t R^t\|^2 + C^+ \sum_{n=1}^{m^+} \xi_n + C^- \sum_{n=1}^{m^-} \xi_n \qquad (3)$$

$$\text{s.t.} \quad \beta^t x_n^+ \geq 1 - \xi_n , \quad \forall x_n^+$$

$$\beta^t x_n^- \leq -1 + \xi_n , \quad \forall x_n^-$$

where the regularization matrix R^t is diagonal. The elements of R^t are positive, such that $R_{ii}^t = \{1, \tau\}$ and $\tau < 1$ attenuates the features outside the down-sampled, canonical segmentation mask of t-th group of examples. The above formulation states that our model β^t should learn to assign scores higher than 1 to positive examples x_n^+ and assign scores lower than -1 to negative examples x_n^-. The objective function penalizes violations of these constraints with slack variables $\xi_n \geq 0$, asymmetrically weighted by constants C^+ and C^-. The negative examples x_n^- come from incorrect detections, which are mined as hard-negatives on images without surgical instruments. We used INRIA pedestrian dataset for this task. We randomly selected 50 images from the dataset when learning each template that amounted to $m^- < 10^4$ negative training examples. Figure 2 (bottom) illustrates some of the learned templates.

The segmentation masks that are representative of each cluster are obtained as a binary sum of example masks. However, some examples may be less similar to other ones in the cluster, unnecessarily widening the canonical segmentation masks. To alleviate this, we use the scores of each positive example after having learned the SVM model for each template in order to compute a weighted average of example segmentation masks. In effect, we obtain a refined canonical segmentation mask for each cluster that we use for segmentation at test-time.

4   Experiments and Results

This section quantitatively (Fig. 4) and qualitatively (Figs. 5 and 6) evaluates the performance of our method in locating parts of robotic instruments.

Dataset. We evaluate the performance of our method on a dataset of three video sequences S1–S3. The sequences show two da Vinci needle drivers that manip-ulate a surgical suture on phantom background [9]. The instruments are always in view. Large shape deformations of the end-effectors are the main challenges of this dataset. The sequences have 613, 904, and 505 frames, respectively, with frame size of 360×640 pixels. We annotated the dataset with four keypoints of the tool parts, shaft ending, center joint, and two forcep tips, and with contours of both tools, which yielded segmentation masks. We trained the detector on the sequence S1 and tested it on the sequences S2 and S3. The training set was augmented to $m^+ \approx 9 \times 10^4$ positive examples by rotating each frame every $5°$ within $180°$ interval, followed by horizontal flipping.

Evaluation protocol. We evaluate our method in two scenarios. After non-maximum suppressing the detections, the protocol evaluates: (i) all detections and (ii) top-2 detections. The first scenario assumes the number of tools in the videos is unknown to the algorithm and reports average precision of keypoints (APK) using standard recall and precision. We also report on the recall of the detector when it knows there are two tools present in the videos. We count a detection as true positive when it is close to the ground truth. The closeness of the detected and ground truth keypoints is evaluated using the KBB metric [6]. The euclidean distance between both points is first normalized by the larger of the sides of the box that tightly bounds all end-effector keypoints, and then compared with α-thresholds. Unmatched ground truth is false negative. To evaluate the segmentation results, we use the DICE metric.

Implementation details. The appearance templates are defined in the feature space of histograms of oriented gradients (HOGs). We set sbin = 8 for the HOG cells and clip histogram magnitudes to 0.2. In order to account for specularities on the tool surface, the feature descriptor only uses 9 absolute orientations of image gradients, bypassing orientation-sensitive cues. The minimal and maximal side size of the learned templates is 6 and 12, respectively. The SVM hyperparameters are asymmetrically set to $C^+ = 10$ and $C^- = 1$ and account for $m^+ \ll m^-$ imbalance in the training set. The regularization parameter in R is set to $\tau = 0.1$.

A pair of training examples is claimed alike when their segmentation masks cross-match to their distance transforms, both satisfying the matching threshold of 300. Setting the threshold to this value yielded ~3500 clusters, an acceptable tradeoff between the number of clusters and their sizes, as shown in Fig. 3. We retain all clusters during learning the templates, even the ones with a single example.

The main part of the algorithm was implemented in Matlab environment, while convolution was implemented in C++ and CUDA. We tested the computational performance of the algorithm on a multicore CPU (Intel Core i7-4930K) with 64 GB RAM and on a GPU (NVIDIA GeForce GTX 780Ti). The timings of four implementation variants are shown in the right part of Fig. 4. Specifically, at test time our tailored GPU-based implementation requires ~0.8 s to detect robotic parts with ~3500 templates in each frame, while an off-the-shelf GPU code[1] requires ~4 s. Training a template proceeds separately from other templates and lends itself to parallelization. Training a single template and ten batches of templates in parallel took less than 2 min and 9 h, respectively.

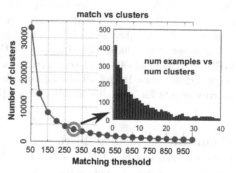

Fig. 3. Matching threshold for grouping binary masks *vs* number of produced clusters. At the threshold 300, there are over 3500 clusters, where 400 clusters have one example (upper right). There is unequal distribution of examples across clusters.

---

[1] Eklund, A., Dufort, P., Non-separable 2D, 3D, and 4D Filtering with CUDA.

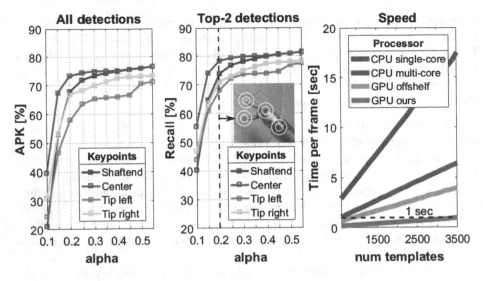

Fig. 4. Quantitative results (best viewed in color). **Left**: Performance of our method in locating four keypoints of da Vinci end-effectors in phantom data setting. The APK and Recall metrics, evaluating all and top-2 detections, respectively, show that locating the tool center is the easiest for our method in both cases. We also show the extent of circular regions at each keypoint, inside which a candidate is counted as true positive. Here, the circles (white) have two rigorous radii that correspond to alpha values of 0.1 and 0.2. **Right**: The computational performance of the algorithm was tested in four variants. Notably, our GPU-based implementation scales evidently better with the number of templates than its both CPU-based counterparts and than off-the-shelf GPU code. For ~3500 templates, it requires ~0.8 s per frame to locate the keypoints of both end-effectors. Both GPU-based convolutions also offer considerable computational improvements for a smaller number of templates. (Color figure online)

Quantitative results. In the task of segmentation of the end-effector, our method achieves the DICE score of 64% and 66% when all and top-2 detections are evaluated, respectively. Moreover, its performance in pose estimation is 67% and 73%, averaged over all four keypoints at threshold $\alpha = 0.2$, for all and top-2 detections, respectively. The obtained results are quite satisfactory and promising given that our templates are trained, on average, only on dozens of positive examples. Further results are shown in Fig. 4.

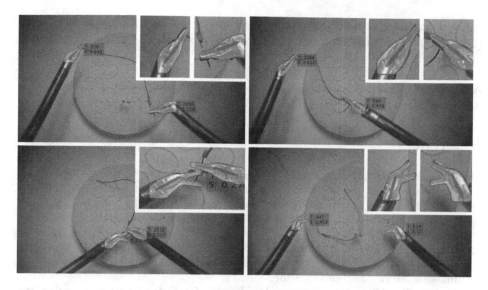

Fig. 5. Correct top-2 detections. Our method has to select the right templates from thousands of potential templates. It can successfully locate robotic parts of multiple instruments and segment the end-effectors at varying scale, articulation, and proximity. The yellow boxes show the type T and the score S of the found templates. (Color figure online)

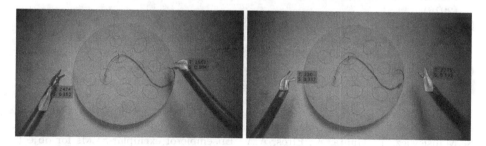

Fig. 6. Analysis of failure cases indicates the method can get confused by the background (here, it slid to the shaft part) and suffers from double-counting errors (right).

5   Conclusion

In this work we proposed a shape-based method for pose estimation of surgical end-effectors. The method groups image examples of the robotic end-effectors by successfully leveraging manually annotated shapes of the end-effectors. The obtained tight appearance clusters allow learning an ensemble of scale-variant and pose-dedicated appearance templates. The templates transfer skeletons and segmentation masks that are specific to particular end-effector articulations. Despite that the tool articulation produces thousands of templates during learning, we achieve frame processing rate below 1 s per frame by convolving the entry image only at its original scale. Our future work will focus on obtaining the segmentation masks automatically in order to learn the template ensemble on-the-fly in unsupervised manner.

Acknowledgment. This work was partially supported by the National Science Center under the agreement UMO-2014/13/D/ST7/03358.

References

1. Allan, M., Chang, P.-L., Ourselin, S., Hawkes, D.J., Sridhar, A., Kelly, J., Stoyanov, D.: Image based surgical instrument pose estimation with multi-class labelling and optical flow. In: Navab, N., Hornegger, J., Wells, W.M., Frangi, A.F. (eds.) MICCAI 2015. LNCS, vol. 9349, pp. 331–338. Springer, Cham (2015). doi:10.1007/978-3-319-24553-9_41
2. Bouget, D., Benenson, R., Omran, M., Riffaud, L., Schiele, B., Jannin, P.: Detecting surgical tools by modelling local appearance and global shape. IEEE Trans. Med. Imaging **34**(12), 2603–2617 (2015)
3. Bouget, D., Allan, M., Stoyanov, D., Jannin, P.: Vision-based and marker-less surgical tool detection and tracking: a review of the literature. Med. Image Anal. **35**, 633–654 (2017)
4. Du, X., Allan, M., Dore, A., Ourselin, S., Hawkes, D., Kelly, J.D., Stoyanov, D.: Combined 2D and 3D tracking of surgical instruments for minimally invasive and robotic-assisted surgery. Int. J. Comput. Assist. Radiol. Surgery **11**(6), 1109–1119 (2016)
5. Hinterstoisser, S., Cagniart, C., Ilic, S., Sturm, P., Navab, N., Fua, P., Lepetit, V.: Gradient response maps for real-time detection of textureless objects. IEEE Trans. Pattern Anal. Mach. Intell. **34**(5), 876–888 (2012)
6. Laina, I., Rieke, N., Rupprecht, C., Vizcano, J. P., Eslami, A., Tombari, F., Navab, N.: Concurrent segmentation and localization for tracking of surgical instruments. arXiv preprint (2017). arXiv:1703.10701
7. Malisiewicz, T., Efros, A.A.: Improving spatial support for objects via multiple segmentations. In: British Machine Vision Conference (2007)
8. Malisiewicz, T., Gupta, A., Efros, A.A.: Ensemble of exemplar-SVMs for object detection and beyond. In: International Conference on Computer Vision, pp. 89–96 (2011)
9. Padoy, N., Hager, G.D.: Deformable tracking of textured curvilinear objects. In: British Machine Vision Conference, pp. 1–11 (2012)
10. Pezzementi, Z., Voros, S., Hager, G.D.: Articulated object tracking by rendering consistent appearance parts. In: IEEE International Conference on Robotics and Automation, pp. 3940–3947 (2009)
11. Reiter, A., Allen, P.K., Zhao, T.: Feature classification for tracking articulated surgical tools. In: Ayache, N., Delingette, H., Golland, P., Mori, K. (eds.) MICCAI 2012. LNCS, vol. 7511, pp. 592–600. Springer, Heidelberg (2012). doi:10.1007/978-3-642-33418-4_73
12. Reiter, A., Allen, P.K., Zhao, T.: Marker-less articulated surgical tool detection. Comput. Assist. Radiol. Surg. (2012)
13. Sarikaya, D., Corso, J., Guru, K.: Detection and localization of robotic tools in robot-assisted surgery videos using deep neural networks for region proposal and detection. IEEE Trans. Med. Imaging **36**, 1542–1549 (2017)

14. Staub, C., Lenz, C., Panin, G., Knoll, A., Bauernschmitt, R.: Contour-based surgical instrument tracking supported by kinematic prediction. In: RAS and EMBS International Conference on Biomedical Robotics and Biomechatronics, pp. 746–752 (2010)
15. Sznitman, R., Becker, C., Fua, P.: Fast part-based classification for instrument detection in minimally invasive surgery. In: Golland, P., Hata, N., Barillot, C., Hornegger, J., Howe, R. (eds.) MICCAI 2014. LNCS, vol. 8674, pp. 692–699. Springer, Cham (2014). doi:10.1007/978-3-319-10470-6_86
16. Wesierski, D., Wojdyga, G., Jezierska, A.: Instrument tracking with rigid part mixtures model. In: Luo, X., Reichl, T., Reiter, A., Mariottini, G.-L. (eds.) CARE 2015. LNCS, vol. 9515, pp. 22–34. Springer, Cham (2016). doi:10.1007/978-3-319-29965-5_3
17. Yang, G.-Z., Cambias, J., Cleary, K., Daimler, E., Drake, J., Dupont, P., Hata, N., Kazanzides, P., Martel, S., et al.: Medical robotics - regulatory, ethical, and legal considerations for increasing levels of autonomy. Sci. Robot. 2(4), eaam8638 (2017)
18. Ye, M., Zhang, L., Giannarou, S., Yang, G.-Z.: Real-time 3D tracking of articulated tools for robotic surgery. In: Ourselin, S., Joskowicz, L., Sabuncu, M.R., Unal, G., Wells, W. (eds.) MICCAI 2016. LNCS, vol. 9900, pp. 386–394. Springer, Cham (2016). doi:10.1007/978-3-319-46720-7_45

3D Endoscope System Using Asynchronously Blinking Grid Pattern Projection for HDR Image Synthesis

Ryo Furukawa[1(✉)], Masahito Naito[1], Daisuke Miyazaki[1], Masahi Baba[1], Shinsaku Hiura[1], Yoji Sanomura[2], Shinji Tanaka[2], and Hiroshi Kawasaki[3]

[1] Hiroshima City University, Hiroshima, Japan
{ryo-f,miyazaki,baba,hiura}@hiroshima-cu.ac.jp,
naito@ime.hiroshima-cu.ac.jp
[2] Hiroshima University Hospital, Hiroshima, Japan
{sanomura,colon}@hiroshima-cu.ac.jp
[3] Kyushu University, Fukuoka, Japan
kawasaki@ait.kyushu-u.ac.jp

Abstract. 3D endoscopic systems have been researched and developed to measure the actual shape and size of living tissues for the purpose of remote surgery and diagnosis, to name a few. For such systems, active stereo that consists of a camera and a pattern projector (*i.e.*, structured light systems) is a promising solution because of simple system with high accuracy. Recently, an active-stereo-based 3D endoscope system has been proposed, in which many practical problems were solved such as shallow focal range of the pattern projector or strong diffusion by living tissues. To use the laser pattern projector for endoscopic systems, two fundamental issues arise; a limited dynamic range of the endoscopic camera and a calibration of the system. In this paper, we proposed a new high dynamic range (HDR) image synthesis technique for a laser pattern projector as well as an auto-calibration technique for dynamic motion. Quantitative experiments are conducted to show the effectiveness of the method followed by a demonstration using real endoscopic system.

1 Introduction

3D endoscopic systems have been intensively researched and developed to measure the actual shape and size of living tissues for the strong demands on remote surgery, diagnosis and so on. For example, in the diagnosis, the size of the tumor is an important factor to decide the stage of cancer. There are several techniques for 3D endoscopic systems, such as binocular stereo, active stereo by projector-camera pair, time of flight, etc. Among them, active stereo is one of the most promising techniques because of its simple configuration, *e.g.*, conventional endoscopic systems can be used without any modification. Although there are several issues to apply active stereo for endoscopic systems, such as dark and shallow focal range of the pattern projector, strong diffusion by tissue, etc., those issues are efficiently solved by a laser pattern projector recently [1,2]. Those systems

© Springer International Publishing AG 2017
M.J. Cardoso et al. (Eds.): CARE/CLIP 2017, LNCS 10550, pp. 16–28, 2017.
DOI: 10.1007/978-3-319-67543-5_2

use a micro-sized pattern projector with diffractive optical element (DOE) and have successfully reconstructed *ex vivo* human tumor samples. However, if we use the system with *in vivo* environment, other fundamental issues will arise; one is insufficient dynamic range of captured image because of the limited size of image sensor under no external light and the other is an unstable calibration of the system because of dynamic motion during an actual endoscopic operation.

In this paper, we proposed a new high dynamic range (HDR) imaging technique for a laser pattern projector as well an auto-calibration technique for dynamic motion. Usually HDR images are synthesized by using multiple-exposure images, however, it is usually impossible to precisely control the exposure of the camera of commonly available endoscopic systems. Therefore, we adopt to vary the intensity of the projector during the operation. In addition, to avoid complicated systems, we use simple signal switching (on-and-off) device without any synchronization mechanism. Multiple exposure images are efficiently captured by frequency difference between the camera and projector's fps. We also propose an auto-calibration technique realized by simultaneous capture of the head of the pattern projector as well as the projected pattern onto the target object. By softly imposing the 2-DOF ambiguity constraint [1], not only 6-DOF extrinsic parameters are robustly estimated, but also scale ambiguity is effectively eliminated.

By using our HDR synthesis technique and auto calibration algorithm, we can achieve an efficient and accurate reconstruction of tissue in metric 3D under practical operation of endoscopic system. In the experiments, we show the effectiveness of our technique with several tests using the real system, and demonstrate the successful reconstruction of the inside of real stomach of pig.

2 Related Work

3D endoscopes based on binocular stereo [3,4] are actively being researched at the present. For the binocular stereo algorithm, which is a typical passive stereo technique, correspondence retrieval is essentially difficult, especially on textureless surfaces. To cope with textureless surfaces, techniques using Shape from Shading (SfS) [5] have been proposed, however, the 3D reconstruction is only up-to-scale and it cannot be directly applied for measuring real sizes of 3D tissues. For laparoscopes for surgery, several structured-light systems have been already proposed [6,7].

An active stereo technique is a simple solution for the aforementioned problems. For example, a single-line laser scanner attached to the scope head was used to measure tissue shape [8]. However, the scope head had to be actuated in a direction parallel to the target, which limited the practical applicability of the technique. Some other vision techniques using special cameras being applied to endoscopes such as ToF sensors [9,10]. However, original resolution of ToF sensor is considerably low [9] or the size is too large and only applicable to laparoscope systems [10]. Recently, we proposed a structured light system for endoscope [1,2,11], which allows users to update a common endoscope system without any reconfiguration. However, there are several problems with the system and our technique can provide practical solution.

One contribution of our technique is HDR image synthesis for endoscopic system. Usually HDR images are synthesized by using multiple-exposure images [12]. However, it is usually difficult to capture images with different exposures using ordinary video cameras. There are several techniques which achieve HDR synthesis and tone-mapping for video [13,14], however active lighting conditions are not considered. If a lighting condition can be precisely controlled with camera synchronization, multi-exposure images are easily retrieved. Though, we assume only on-and-off controllable pattern projector with no synchronization mechanism, and there is no paper has published yet of such an approach.

In terms of auto-calibration, tons of techniques are proposed for binocular stereo so far [15]. However, there is a few techniques for active stereo systems, especially for structured light systems [16,17]. It should be noted that scale ambiguity remains for common auto-calibration techniques and should be solved for endoscopic systems.

3   DOE-Based Laser Pattern Projector for Endoscopy

3.1   System Configuration

A projector-camera system is constructed by installing a micro pattern projector on a standard endoscope as shown in Fig. 1(a). For our system, we used a FujiFilm VP-4450HD system coupled with a EG-590WR scope. The DOE-based laser pattern projector is inserted in the endoscope through the instrument channel, the projector protrudes slightly from the endoscope head and emits structured light. The light source of the projector is a green laser module with a wavelength of 517 nm. The laser light is transmitted through a single-mode optical fiber to the head of the DOE projector. The DOE generates the pattern through diffraction of the laser light. The 3D measurements are conducted by structured light method with the projector-camera pair composed of the single endoscope camera and the pattern projector.

Our system is based on active stereo method that we have proposed [2], in which a gap-based grid pattern is used for avoiding effect of subsurface scattering that is harmful for 3D reconstruction. The projected pattern consists of only line segments as shown in Fig. 1(c) (top). The vertical lines of pattern are all connected and straight, whereas the horizontal segments are designed in a way to leave a small variable vertical gap between adjacent horizontal segments and their intersections with the same vertical line. With this configuration, a higher-level ternary code emerges from the design with the following three codewords: S (the end-points of both sides have the same height), L (the end-point of the left side is higher), and R (the end-point of the left side is higher). The codes of the pattern of Fig. 1(c) (top) are shown by color in Fig. 1(c) (bottom).

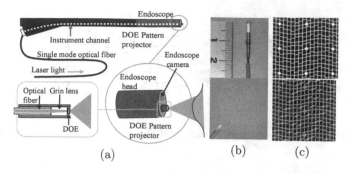

(a) (b) (c)

Fig. 1. System configuration: (a) System components. (b) DOE micro projector. (c) The projected pattern(top), and embedded codewords of S colored in red, L in blue, and R in green (bottom). S means edges of the left and the right sides have the same height, L means the left side is higher, and R means the right is higher. (Color figure online)

3.2 3D Reconstruction

The source image is first geometrically corrected on the fish-eye lens distortion. Noises of the image are suppressed using Gaussian filters or median filters at the same time. The projected vertical and horizontal lines are detected in the undistorted image using the line detection algorithm from Sagawa *et al.* [18]. This method can detect projected parallel lines whose approximate directions are known, ignoring intersecting non-vertical lines, based on loopy belief propagation.

From the detected line patterns, grid-graph structure is constructed by detecting intersections between the horizontal and vertical lines. Then, each node is connected with its up, down, left, or right adjacent nodes by vertical or horizontal edges. Some horizontal edges might have a missing edge because of misdetection. In this case, the node will only have either a left or a right edge, which may be later matched by looking at other connectivity of the grid graph. Figures 8(f) and 9(b)(f) show examples of the detected vertical and horizontal patterns with estimated gap codes.

Let the detected grid-graph be G, and let the grid-graph of the pattern in Fig. 1(c) be P. Note that graph G may lack some edges, or have undesired false edges, missing labels, or false labels of $S/L/R$ as shown in the left part of Fig. 2.

To match G and P allowing topological errors, we exploit the notion of local sub-graph patterns (LSGPs). We define an LSGP to be a sub-graph of a grid-graph used as a template for matching common local topologies of G and P (in Fig. 2, the left part shows G, the right part shows P, and the middle part shows LSGPs). Given a dictionary of LSGPs, G may be matched to P robustly to missing or false edges. By providing multiple LSGPs and trying to match G and P using each of them, flexible matching can be realized. In our implementation, an LSGP is represented by a path that traces all of its edges. To merge all the matching results of LSGPs, voting is used.

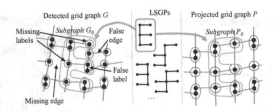

Fig. 2. Matching the detected grid graph and the projected pattern using LSGPs.

Once the correspondence of the captured image to the pattern is obtained, the points on the vertical and horizontal lines are reconstructed in 3D using a light-sectioning method.

4   Auto-Calibration of the Projector Position

In this system, the target surface, which is projected by pattern projector, is captured by the endoscope camera. Since the head of the projector is not tightly fixed to the endoscope, the relative position between the projector head and the endoscopic camera varies during endoscopic operations, such as bending the head. Since, for active stereo techniques, the position of the projector is an important parameter for 3D reconstruction, such unstable condition is problematic for robust and accurate shape measurement.

Furukawa *et al.* [1] modeled the relative position by 2-DOF rigid transformation, where projector translates along or rotates around the axis of the instrument channel. This 2-DOF model could be applied to our system if the pattern projector's outer diameter perfectly fitted to the inner diameter of the instrument channel. However, there should be some margin between the projector and the channel, for the projector to be inserted during the endoscopic operations. In real situations, the projector have more freedom to move beyond the 2-DOF model within the margin.

Another problem of work of Furukawa *et al.* [1] is that they estimate the projector's position by detecting a marker drawn on the projector from the endoscope image. In real situations where endoscope image is captured in dark environments, markers drawn on the projector are difficult to detect from the captured images.

In the proposed system, we use silhouette of the projector and the markers embedded in the grid pattern projected onto the target surface. The silhouette of the projector can be observed from the captured image, even if there are not illumination except for the projected pattern. The markers in the grid pattern can be also detected from the same image (see Fig. 8(d) for an example, where the projector silhouette can be observed at the bottom of the image).

The actual process is as follows: From the input image captured for measurement, markers in the grid pattens (m_i) are detected. Also, several points in the projector's silhouette (s_j) are also sampled (Fig. 3). Note that, we can

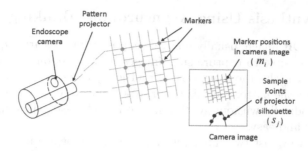

Fig. 3. Input points for auto-calibration of the projector.

assume epipolar geometries fullilled between the endoscope camera and the pattern projector, if the estimated parameters are correct for the auto-calibration. Since a pattern projector can be modeled in the same way as a camera, epipolar geometries can be used for a projector-camera pair.

The auto-calibration is processed as an optimization of 6-DOF rigind transformation parameters that represent projector's position. Here, we devide the estimated 6 parameters into 2 sets of parameters: one set is for 2-DOF freedom described in [1] and the other is for the rest 4 parameters. We regard the 2-DOF parameters as freely changing parameters, since they represent the motion of the pattern projector that rotates around and translates along the axis of the instrument channel, while we supress the rest 4 parameters since they are deviation from the 2-DOF freedom of [1]. Because of this 'soft' 2-DOF constraint, the estimated projector position does not have scale ambiguity.

The optimized cost function is defined as follows:

1. The cost function takes 6 parameters $p_1, p_2, q_1, q_2, q_3, q_4$, representing the 3D position of the projector (rotation $\mathbf{R}$ and translation $\mathbf{t}$) relative to the endoscope camera, where p_1 and p_2 are 2-DOF parameters described in [1], and $q_1, \cdots, q_4$ represents the rest of the fill 6-DOF rigid transformation that should be supressed.
2. For the markers m_i, the corresponding epipolar line is calculated, and the distance between m_i and the epipolar line is calculated as g_i.
3. The virtual silhouette of the projector is rendered as a cylinder moved by the rigid transformation $\mathbf{R}$ and $\mathbf{t}$. From each s_j, the minimum distance from s_j to contours of the rendered silhouette is calculated as h_j.
4. $\sum_i (g_i)^2 + w_1 \sum_j (h_j)^2 + w_2 \sum_k (q_k)^2$ is calculated as the cost value, where w_1 is weight of the cost of silhouette fitting and w_2 is weight for supresson of the parameters representing the deviation from the 2-DOF freedom [1].

In current implementation, selection of the marker position and sampling points on the silhouette contour are conducted manually for each frame in image sequences and auto-calibration should be conducted for each frame. Further automation for point selection will be our future work.

5   HDR Synthesis Using Asynchronous Blinking Pattern

To synthesize HDR image, usually multiple-exposure images are required. However, it is not possible to capture such images with commonly available endoscopic systems. To solve the issue, we control the light source instead of the camera, *i.e.*, blinking the pattern in this paper. Note that we just switch the pattern on-and-off periodically without synchronization mechanism, such an implementation is simple and easy.

The reason why just two intensities for the projector are fine to synthesize HDR whereas usually multiple exposures are required, is based on the difference of frequency of the camera and the projector. Suppose n Hz for the camera and m Hz for the projector. Usually video mode of camera is set burst mode, *i.e.*, the shutter is always open, and the shutter speed is $1/n$ sec. On the other hand, switching (on-and-off) signal makes half of exposure time, *i.e.*, $1/(2m)$ for the projector. Then the exposure time is $1/(2m) - s$, when the offset is $s (s < 1/(2m)$, $n < 2m)$. Since s varies at each capture because of the frequency difference, exposure time is also changed at each capture as shown in Fig. 4. For example, if $n = 30$ and $m = 26$, then exposure time varies approximately with 8 Hz and we can synthesize HDR using the 8 frames. Then, tone mapping is applied to the HDR images to make 8bit images, which allows to use conventional image processing tools.

To make HDR, exposure time is supposed to be known. If the camera and the projector are synchronized, the s is known and an exact exposure time can be calculated. However, it requires a complicated device to achieve synchronization. To avoid such additional devices, we estimate the exposure time only from captured images. In our implementation, we simply average the intensity of the pattern excluding outliers with simple thresholding technique for each frame and use the ratio of the average as for the ratio of exposure time.

Normally, multiple-exposure for HDR image synthesis is conducted for a static camera and the scene. Since the endoscope and the target tissue can be move, they are not static. However, for the above setup of $n = 30$ and $m = 26$, we can obtain a image set of around 8 different exposure in $1/4$ s, which is short enough to assume the camera and the scene is static if we hold the endoscope still.

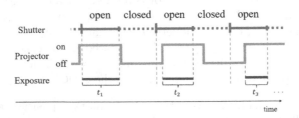

Fig. 4. Relationship between a shutter speed and a pattern projection time: t_i represents an exposure time.

6 Experiments

6.1 Improvement Using HDR Image for 3D Reconstruction

To show effectiveness of the HDR image generation, we tested our algorithm using a human hand as the target object. We first captured images of the target surface which is projected by a blinking laser pattern projector. Although pattern is just illuminated bright and dark repeatedly, we could obtain an image sequence with different exposures. We have extarcted 8 images of one multi-exposure cycle $I_1, I_2, \cdots I_8$. I_1, I_3, I_5 and I_7 are shown in Fig. 5. With our HDR image synthesis method, image sequence of single period of intensity change is automatically extracted by finding the darkest frame in three consecutive frames; Fig. 5 is one of such sequence.

Then, HDR image is created from the sequence, and then, tone-mapped for 3D reconstructed algorithm. The HDR image is shown in Fig. 6(b). The 3D reconstructed results with/without HDR algorithm are shown in Fig. 6(c) and (d). The numbers of reconstructed points for each frame and HDR image are shown in Fig. 7. From Fig. 7, we can confirm that the area that was successfully reconstructed from the HDR image was larger than the results of the any of the original input images. In Fig. 6, we can see that the regions around the brightest center marker were reconstructed in the result of I_T (HDR image), whereas, in

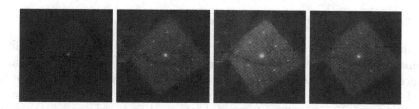

Fig. 5. Original images: I_1, I_3, I_5, I_7 from 8 images $I_1, I_2, \cdots, I_8$. Note that the exposure was changing frame by frame.

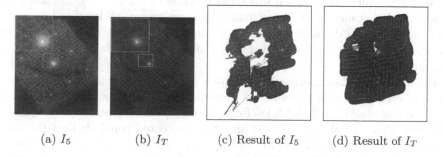

(a) I_5 (b) I_T (c) Result of I_5 (d) Result of I_T

Fig. 6. Comparison between the original and the tone-mapped HDR images. (a) I_5 from Fig. 5, which was most successfully reconstructed in images I_1 to I_8. (b) The tone-mapped HDR image generated from I_1 to I_8. (c) 3D reconstruction result of (a). (d) 3D reconstruction result of (b).

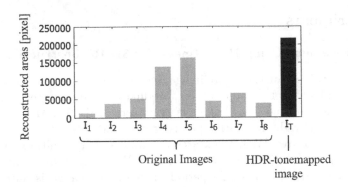

Fig. 7. Comparison of 3D reconstructed areas of original and tone-mapped HDR images.

the result of I_5 (note that I_5 was the most successfully reconstructed image from Fig. 7), the same regions were not reconstructed. In Fig. 6, we can also see that the noises in the source images are reduced in the tone-mapped HDR image, because multiple images are merged so that independent noises are suppressed. From the results, we have confirmed that HDR image enhanced the image quality and reduced the negative effects of over and under exposures and noises.

6.2   3D Reconstruction Inside Stomach of a Pig

To evaluate the system in more realistic conditions, we captured shapes inside a stomach of a pig, which is often used for evaluation purpose and practice of endoscopists. To evaluate the scales captured by the 3D endoscope, we first curved several markers on the surface of pig's stomach, then, reconstruct 3D shape of the entire surface. The distances between the two markers are estimated and compared to the ground truth, which is obtained by measuring the real distances between the markers after the measurement process; we cut and opened the stomach. Since the stomach was inflated while the endoscopy diagnosis, the ground truth distances that are actually measured were considered to be smaller than the estimated distance with our technique. To compensate such error, we also measure the ground truth distance while expanding the stomach surface manually.

Figure 8 shows the experimental situation and the measurement results. Comparison between estimated results and ground truth are shown in Table 1. The precision was about 5.0% and 2.1% from the unexpanded ground truth. Considering the difference of measurement situation, we could conclude that the measurement was sufficiently accurate. In Fig. 8(g) and (h), we also show the result of auto-calibration. In Fig. 8(g), which shows situation before auto-calibration, the rendered silhouette of the projector is different from the captured silhouette of Fig. 8(e). After auto-calibration shown in Fig. 8(h), the projector position fits to the captured image, and the epipolar lines lie on the marker position.

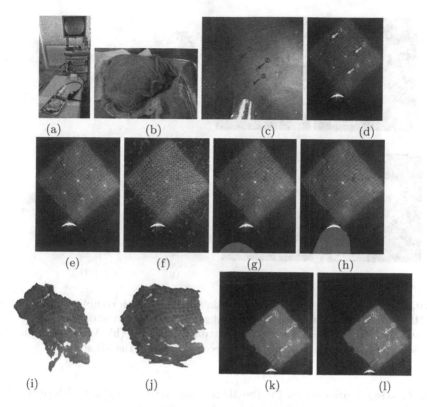

Fig. 8. 3D reconstruction of bio-tissue inside a pig stomach with markers. (a) The environment of the experiment. (b) The pig-stomach cut open after experiment session. (c) The appearance inside the stomach with marker positions. (d) The captured image with the pattern projected. (e) The HDR enhanced image. (f) The detected grid graph. (g), (h) Before and after the auto-calibration of the projector. The rendered projector positing is the read cylinder and the epipolar lines are pink line segments. (g) is before the auto-calibration and (h) is after the auto-calibration. (i), (j) Reconstructed 3D shape rendered from two different view points. (k), (l) Distance measurements between the two markers. Red regions are reconstructed areas. (Color figure online)

Table 1. Estimated distances between two markers of pig stomach

Marker IDs	Ground Truth	Ground Truth (expanded)	Our result
1 and 2	24.6 mm	29.4 mm	25.9 mm
2 and 3	14.2 mm	15.1 mm	13.9 mm

While measuring the pig's stomach, we also measured more complicated shapes such as ridges on the surface. Figure 9 shows examples of the captured images and the reconstructed shapes. We can confirm that the ridges or concaves

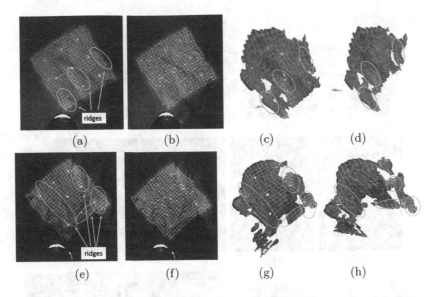

(a)   (b)   (c)   (d)

(e)   (f)   (g)   (h)

Fig. 9. 3D reconstruction of bio-tissue inside a stomach with complicated shapes. (a) The HDR processed input image. (b) The detected grid graph with codes. (c)(d) The reconstructed shapes viewed from different directions. (e)–(h) Another result. Note that ridges of the surface are successfully reconstructed in the 3D shape.

of the bio-tissues are captured in the 3D reconstruction results, which proves that our technique can recover dense shape of complicated surfaces.

7   Conclusion

We proposed a 3D endoscopic system based on an active stereo, where the laser pattern projector consists of a DOE that generates a special line-based grid pattern. Since the laser projector has a strong light intensity and dynamic range of the camera is not enough, we propose a new HDR image synthesis technique using a blinking modulation applied to the projector. In addition, the head of endoscope dynamically moves during an actual operation, and thus, the relative position of a camera and a projector is not fixed with respect to each other. Since the relative position should be known for 3D reconstruction, we propose an auto-calibration technique using the silhouette of the pattern projector. The ability of the techniques were confirmed by intensive experiments using real endoscopic systems and demonstrated by reconstructing the 3D shape of the inside surface of a pig's stomach. Our future work is to construct the realtime system and use it to actual diagnosis and operations.

References

1. Furukawa, R., Masutani, R., Miyazaki, D., Baba, M., Hiura, S., Visentini-Scarzanella, M., Morinaga, H., Kawasaki, H., Sagawa, R.: 2-dof auto-calibration for a 3D endoscope system based on active stereo. In: 2015 37th Annual International Conference of the IEEE Engineering in Medicine and Biology Society (EMBC), pp. 7937–7941, August 2015
2. Furukawa, R., Sanomura, Y., Tanaka, S., Yoshida, S., Sagawa, R., Visentini-Scarzanella, M., Kawasaki, H.: 3D endoscope system using doe projector. In: The 38th Annual International Conference of the IEEE Engineering in Medicine and Biology Society (EMBC 2016) (2016)
3. Nagakura, T., Michida, T., Hirao, M., Kawahara, K., Yamada, K.: The study of three-dimensional measurement from an endoscopic images with stereo matching method. In: Automation Congress, 2006. WAC 2006. World, pp. 1–4, July 2006
4. Stoyanov, D., Scarzanella, M.V., Pratt, P., Yang, G.-Z.: Real-time stereo reconstruction in robotically assisted minimally invasive surgery. In: Jiang, T., Navab, N., Pluim, J.P.W., Viergever, M.A. (eds.) MICCAI 2010. LNCS, vol. 6361, pp. 275–282. Springer, Heidelberg (2010). doi:10.1007/978-3-642-15705-9_34
5. Visentini-Scarzanella, M., Stoyanov, D., Yang, G.: Metric depth recovery from monocular images using shape-from-shading and specularities. In: ICIP, Orlando, USA, pp. 25–28 (2012)
6. Maurice, X., Albitar, C., doignon, C., de Mathelin, M.: A structured light-based laparoscope with real-time organs' surface reconstruction for minimally invasive surgery. In: 2012 Annual International Conference of the IEEE Engineering in Medicine and Biology Society, pp. 5769–5772, August 2012
7. Reiter, A., Sigaras, A., Fowler, D., Allen, P.K.: Surgical structured light for 3D minimally invasive surgical imaging. In: 2014 IEEE/RSJ International Conference on Intelligent Robots and Systems, pp. 1282–1287, September 2014
8. Grasa, O., Bernal, E., Casado, S., Gil, I., Montiel, J.: Visual slam for handheld monocular endoscope. IEEE Trans. Med. Imaging 33(1), 135–146 (2014)
9. Köhler, T., Haase, S., Bauer, S., Wasza, J., Kilgus, T., Maier-Hein, L., Feußner, H., Hornegger, J.: ToF meets RGB: novel multi-sensor super-resolution for hybrid 3-D endoscopy. In: Mori, K., Sakuma, I., Sato, Y., Barillot, C., Navab, N. (eds.) MICCAI 2013. LNCS, vol. 8149, pp. 139–146. Springer, Heidelberg (2013). doi:10.1007/978-3-642-40811-3_18
10. Penne, J., Schaller, C., Engelbrecht, R., Maier-Hein, L., Schmauss, B., Meinzer, H.P., Hornegger, J.: Laparoscopic quantitative 3D endoscopy for image guided surgery. In: Bildverarbeitung für die Medizin, Citeseer, pp. 16–20 (2010)
11. Furukawa, R., Aoyama, M., Hiura, S., Aoki, H., Kominami, Y., Sanomura, Y., Yoshida, S., Tanaka, S., Sagawa, R., Kawasaki, H.: Calibration of a 3d endoscopic system based on active stereo method for shape measurement of biological tissues and specimen. In: EMBC, pp. 4991–4994 (2014)
12. Debevec, P.E., Malik, J.: Recovering high dynamic range radiance maps from photographs. In: SIGGRAPH 2008, pp. 1–10. ACM, New York (2008)
13. Kalantari, N.K., Shechtman, E., Barnes, C., Darabi, S., Goldman, D.B., Sen, P.: Patch-based high dynamic range video. ACM Trans. Graph. 32(6), 202–1 (2013)
14. Eilertsen, G., Mantiuk, R., Unger, J.: A comparative review of tone-mapping algorithms for high dynamic range video. In: Computer Graphics Forum, vol. 36, pp. 565–592. Wiley Online Library (2017)

15. Forsyth, D., Ponce, J.: Computer Vision: A Modern Approach, 2nd edn. Pearson Education Inc., London (2011)
16. Furukawa, R., Kawasaki, H.: Laser range scanner based on self-calibration techniques using coplanarities and metric constraints. Comput. Vis. Image Underst. **113**(11), 1118–1129 (2009)
17. Furukawa, R., Kawasaki, H.: Self-calibration of multiple laser planes for 3D scene reconstruction. In: 3DPVT, pp. 200–207 (2006)
18. Sagawa, R., Ota, Y., Yagi, Y., Furukawa, R., Asada, N., Kawasaki, H.: Dense 3D reconstruction method using a single pattern for fast moving object. In: ICCV (2009)

Towards Real-Time Polyp Detection in Colonoscopy Videos: Adapting Still Frame-Based Methodologies for Video Sequences Analysis

Quentin Angermann[1], Jorge Bernal[2(✉)], Cristina Sánchez-Montes[3],
Maroua Hammami[1], Gloria Fernández-Esparrach[3], Xavier Dray[1,4],
Olivier Romain[1], F. Javier Sánchez[2], and Aymeric Histace[1]

[1] ETIS Lab, ENSEA, University of Cergy-Pontoise, CNRS, Cergy, France
{quentin.angermann,maroua.hammami,
olivier.romain,aymeric.histace}@ensea.fr
[2] Computer Vision Center, Universitat Autonoma de Barcelona, Barcelona, Spain
{jorge.bernal,javier.sanchez}@cvc.uab.cat
[3] Digestive Endoscopy Unit, Hospital Clinic de Barcelona, Barcelona, Spain
{crsanchez,mgfernan}@clinic.cat
[4] St. Antoine Hospital, APHP, Paris, France
xavier.dray@aphp.fr

Abstract. Colorectal cancer is the second cause of cancer death in United States: precursor lesions (polyps) detection is key for patient survival. Though colonoscopy is the gold standard screening tool, some polyps are still missed. Several computational systems have been proposed but none of them are used in the clinical room mainly due to computational constraints. Besides, most of them are built over still frame databases, decreasing their performance on video analysis due to the lack of output stability and not coping with associated variability on image quality and polyp appearance. We propose a strategy to adapt these methods to video analysis by adding a spatio-temporal stability module and studying a combination of features to capture polyp appearance variability. We validate our strategy, incorporated on a real-time detection method, on a public video database. Resulting method detects all polyps under real time constraints, increasing its performance due to our adaptation strategy.

Keywords: Polyp detection · Colonoscopy · Real time · Spatio temporal coherence

1 Introduction

Colorectal cancer (CRC) is the second leading cause of cancer death in United States, causing about 49,190 deaths during 2016 [1]. CRC's early diagnose is crucial for patient's survival, as precursor lesions (known as polyps) may degenerate into cancer over time. Several techniques have been proposed for lesion screening,

M.J. Cardoso et al. (Eds.): CARE/CLIP 2017, LNCS 10550, pp. 29–41, 2017.
DOI: 10.1007/978-3-319-67543-5_3

such as Wireless Capsule Endoscopy (WCE) or Virtual Colonoscopy (VC) but colonoscopy is still considered as the gold standard tool as it can detect lesions of any size (contrary to VC) and it allows lesion detection and removal during the same procedure (contrary to WCE). Nevertheless, colonoscopy has its own drawbacks being the most relevant of them polyp miss-rate, reported to be up to 22% for the case of small size or flat polyps [10].

Three types of approaches have been tackled to overcome these drawbacks: (1) improvement of endoscopic devices (magnification endoscopes [6]), (2) the development of new imaging technologies such as virtual chromoendoscopy [7,12] and (3) the proposal of computational support systems for colonoscopy aiming to support clinicians during/after the procedure.

Regarding computational systems, several efforts have already tackled automatic polyp detection in colonoscopy videos, ranging from classical hand-crafted shape-based methods [4] to pure machine learning approaches [2,8]. Recently, trending techniques such as deep convolutional networks have been also proposed [13,14] and a comparison between a large number of them was presented in [5] in the context of a global polyp detection challenge.

Despite the large number of approaches, none of them, to the best of our knowledge, are currently used in the exploration room due to: (1) not meeting real-time constraints, (2) not being tested on full length colonoscopy procedures and (3) being developed using still frame data (as fully public annotated video databases are not available). Regarding the latter, development over still frame data present the following problems associated to video analysis: absence of temporal coherence in method output and lack of adaption to higher variability in structures appearance (polyps and other elements) and image quality.

We present in this paper a methodology to adapt existing still-frame based polyp detection methods to video analysis. Our strategy consists of the addition of a spatio-temporal coherence module to stabilize methods output and the combination of different feature types to capture polyp appearance variability throughout a video. We integrate our strategy over an real-time polyp detection method [2]; the whole methodology is validated over a fully publicly annotated video database [3]. This validation is performed using a set of performance metrics chosen to fully represent method performance.

The structure of the rest of this paper is as follows. Section 2 introduces the adaptation strategy as well as the reference polyp detection method. In Sect. 3 we detail the experimental setup, results of which are shown in Sect. 4. We discuss in-depth the performance of the proposed methodology in Sect. 5. We finally the main conclusions of this study are drawn in Sect. 6.

2   Method

2.1   Reference Real-Time Still Frame-Based Polyp Detection Method

As explained in Sect. 1, we will use as reference method the one proposed in [2] which offers a good tradeoff between performance and associated processing time (0.039 ms, meeting real-time constrains over 25 fps videos). This active learning

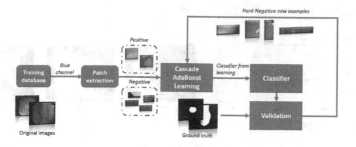

Fig. 1. Still-frame processing pipeline

methodology consists of two different stages: (i) a Cascade AdaBoost learning step for the computation of a classifier, and (ii) a strengthening strategy based on active learning principle using Hard Negative examples [16]. Active learning is used to reinforce the classification performance by adding new negative examples produced by the initial classifier to the learning database.

This initial classifier is trained using six patches from each image of the training database (CVC-ClinicDB [4]): one positive patch covering completely the polyp and five negative ones without any polyp content. We use the Cascade Adaboost strategy (10 stages, with for each of them a targeted true positive rate of 99% and a false positive rate of 50%) to obtain this initial classifier, which is tested as a polyp detector function on each of the images of the complete dataset. As a result, the classifier provides a set of regions of interest (RoIs) where it predicts polyp presence. We compare prediction results over ground truth; all RoIs that do not contain a polyp are fed into the learning process as hard negative training patches so a new Cascade Adaboost classifier is created. An overview of the full processing training/learning scheme is shown Fig. 1. This process is repeated several times to obtain an optimal performance level. The interested reader can find a full description of the methodology at [2].

2.2 Combination of Feature Types

The use of texture-based descriptors (Local Binary Patterns) was proposed in [2] due the polyp appeared different enough from its surroundings due to the good selection of polyp shots from the corresponding videos. Unfortunately, in full video analysis, the number of false alarms grow due to variations in image quality and polyp appearance and due to the presence of other endoluminal scene elements which can deviate detectors' attention from the polyp.

The reference method allows an straightforward aggregation of other features to complement LBP though it is important to consider the potential impact in computational time of these new features. We propose to combine LBP with Haar features [11] because of the following two reasons: first, they can be fastly computed by using the usual "integral image strategy". Second, they can offer complementary information to LBP in a way such if LBP are more sensitive to the gradient information inside an image, Haar, by computing contrast/homogeneity parameter, can be related to geometrical local properties of a given RoI.

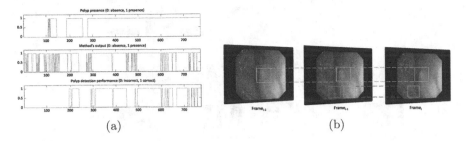

(a)   (b)

Fig. 2. Spatio-temporal coherence module: (a) Example of spatio temporal instability in the output of still frame polyp detection methods when applied on full sequences. (b) Graphical explanation of the proposed solution: Green boxes represent the output in the current frame, blue boxes represents outputs in the previous frames. Green dashed lines connect similar RoIs in consecutive frames (kept in method output) whereas red ones represent unconnected RoIs between consecutive frames (removed in the output). (Color figure online)

2.3 Spatio-Temporal Coherence Module

One big drawback of the use of still-frame based methods for video analysis is that, by default, they do not consider information of previous frames to determine the output of the current ones. Due to this, a given method can show a performance like the one shown in Fig. 2(a) where we can observe that the method is not able to provide a stable output between consecutive frames.

To mitigate this, we propose the decision tree shown in Fig. 3. It is important to mention that to calculate the initial output for a given frame we first perform intra-frame block fusion to only provide as output candidates those RoIs where more individual outputs have been provided by the classifier. Once this is done, when calculating the final output for a given frame, the system considers also the RoIs provided by the classifier in the two previous frames in a way such if RoIs from the previous frame overlap with RoIs provided for the actual frame, these RoIs are kept to generate the final output. If it is not the case, those RoIs without spatio-temporal overlap are not included in the final output.

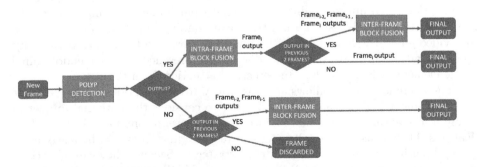

Fig. 3. Decision tree implemented to warrantee spatio-temporal coherence in method output

Table 1. Statistics of CVC-ClinicVideoDB database. PF stands for polyp frames, NPF for non-polyp frames and Paris represents morphology of the polyp according to Paris classification (0-Is for sessile polyps, 0-Ip for pedunculated polyps and 0-IIa for flat-elevated polyps).

Video	PF	NPF	Paris	Video	PF	NPF	Paris	Video	PF	NPF	Paris
1	386	112	0-Is	7	338	103	0-Is	13	620	4	0-Is
2	597	176	0-Is	8	405	44	0-IIa	14	2015	45	0-Is
3	819	153	0-Is	9	532	19	0-Ip	15	360	215	0-Is
4	350	40	0-Is	10	762	78	0-IIa	16	366	5	0-Is
5	412	78	0-Is	11	370	130	0-Is	17	651	146	0-IIa
6	522	335	0-Ip	12	261	124	0-IIa	18	259	122	0-Ip

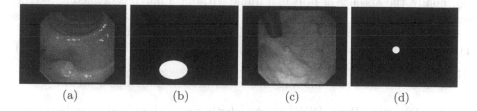

(a)   (b)   (c)   (d)

Fig. 4. Examples of (a, c) original image and (b, d) associated ground truth.

3 Experimental Setup

3.1 Validation Database

We validate our complete methodology over the first fully publicly available video annotated database (CVC-ClinicVideoDB) database, which comprises 18 different standard definition video sequences all showing a polyp. These sequences have been recorded using OLYMPUS QF190 endoscopes and Exera III videograbber. CVC-ClinicVideoDB contains 10924 frames of size 768 × 576, of which 9221 contain a polyp. Table 1 shows statistics of each of the videos of CVC-ClinicVideoDB, including Paris morphology [9] of the different polyps. Ground truth for each frame corresponds to a binary image in which white pixels correspond to polyp pixels in the image (images without polyps do not have any white pixels). CVC-ClinicVideoDB ground truth consists of an ellipse approximating polyp boundary. We show some examples of original images and their corresponding ground truth in Fig. 4.

3.2 Performance Metrics

Before defining the different metrics used to assess method performance, it is worth to mention that the output of the method for a particular frame consist of a series of bounding boxes representing the different RoIs provided by the classifier.

Following guidelines depicted in [5], we will use as first indication of correct detection (True Positive, TP) if the centroid of the RoI falls within the polyp mask. As in this first version of the database we provide ellipses for a weak labelling of the polyp, we have incorporated two additional criteria to determine a TP: (1) having pixel-wise precision within the RoI is higher than 50% (to cover the case of very big polyps against an small RoI) or (2) having a small distance to the centroid of the RoI to the border of the ground truth mask or a pixel-wise recall higher than 50% (to cover the case of small polyps enclosed within a large ground truth area). It is important to mention that we will only account one TP per polyp region in the image, no matter how many RoIs detect it. In case a polyp in a frame is not detected, we have a False Negative (FN) - we can have as many FNs as polyps in the image -. RoIs without overlap with a polyp region are accounted as False Positives (FP) - there can be more than one FP per image - and, finally, the absence of RoIs in a frame without a polyp is defined as a True Negative (TN).

From these definitions, we can calculate the following aggregation metrics: (1) Precision ($Prec = 100 * \frac{TP}{TP+FP}$), (2) Recall ($Rec = 100 * \frac{TP}{TP+FN}$) and (3) F1-score ($F1 = \frac{2*Prec*Rec}{Prec+Rec}$).

We also calculate the following metrics to account for clinical usability:

- Polyp Detection Rate (PDR) checks whether a method is able to detect the polyp at least once in a sequence, following guidelines depicted in [15].
- Mean Processing Time per frame (MPT). Considering videos are recorded at 25 fps, 40 milliseconds is the maximum time processing of a new frame can take to avoid delaying the intervention. MPT includes both frame processing time as well as displaying the results on the monitor.
- Mean Number of False Positives per frame (MNFP).
- Reaction Time (RT) represents the delay (in frames and seconds considering a frame rate of 25fps) between first appearance of the polyp in the sequence and the first correct detection provided by the method [4].

4 Results

4.1 Quantitative Results

We present quantitative results in Table 2, broken down by the different aspects we wanted to test in the study (impact of adaptation strategy, computational efficiency). Before introducing a breakdown of the results, it is important to mention that, as the methodology over which we have incorporated our adaptation strategy incorporates strengthening stages, we will distinguish each strengthening iteration with a cardinal index starting by 0 in a way such classifier Ni will refer to a classifier computed with i strengthening steps.

The first important result to be extracted from Table 2 is that the methodology is able to detect all different polyps in the different sequences at least in one frame, using the same definition proposed in [15]. The basic configuration of the system, as presented in [2], achieves the smallest reaction time.

Table 2. Overall performance results.

Method	PDR	MPT	MNFP	Prec	Rec	F1	RT
Impact of the type of feature descriptor used							
LBPN0	100%	140ms	3.5	12.42%	54.65%	20.24%	7.2 [0.3 sec]
HaarN0	100%	24ms	1.4	23.29%	46.82%	31.10%	17.5 [0.7 sec]
Impact of spatio-temporal coherence (STC)							
LBPN0 noSTC	100%	140ms	3.5	12.42%	54.65%	20.24%	7.2 [0.3 sec]
LBPN0	100%	140ms	1.9	16.25%	41.25%	23.31%	35.0 [1.4 sec]
HaarN0 noSTC	100%	24ms	1.4	23.29%	46.82%	31.10%	17.5 [0.7 sec]
HaarN0	100%	36ms	0.9	27.02%	39.61%	32.12%	38.3 [1.5 sec]
Impact of network strengthening							
LBPN0	100%	140ms	1.9	16.25%	41.25%	23.31%	35.0 [1.4 sec]
LBPN1	100%	160ms	1.1	27.11%	46.02%	34.12%	43.7 [1.7 sec]
LBPN2	100%	162ms	0.7	29.88%	34.96%	32.22%	45.9 [1.8 sec]
HaarN0	100%	36ms	0.9	27.02%	39.61%	32.12%	38.3 [1.5 sec]
HaarN1	100%	21ms	0.6	39.14%	42.56%	40.78%	27.3 [1.1 sec]
Impact of feature aggregation)							
LBPN2	100%	162ms	0.7	29.88%	34.96%	32.22%	45.9 [1.8 sec]
HaarN1	100%	21ms	0.6	39.14%	42.56%	40.78%	27.3 [1.1 sec]
Aggregation	100%	185ms	1.1	30.39%	52.40%	38.47%	15.0 [0.6 sec]

With respect of *the type of features used*, we can observe a positive difference associated to the use of Haar features which leads to a great reduction in the number of false positives while keeping real-time constraints and a similar recall (higher F1-score). LBP offers a slower processing time (140 ms per image) and an excessive number of false alarms (around 3.5 FP per image), which makes its use not compatible with a clinical use.

We broke down the results according to polyp morphology, under the assumption that Haar features should perform better for those types in which the contour can be clearly observed. We present results of this side experiment in Table 3. On the one hand, we can observe how LBP achieves a higher F1-score for flat polyps (higher recall for a similar precision); we associate Haar's worse performance to the lack of strong contours. In this case, LBP takes advantage of the difference in pattern between polyp and mucosa. On the other hand, for peduncular polyps in which their contours are clearly recognizable, we can observe a clearly superior performance of Haar in all performance metrics, especially with respect to RT (difference of more than 3.5 s with respect to LBP).

The use of our *spatio-temporal coherence* module results on an improvement in the overall performance for both descriptors, decreasing in a significant way the average number of FPs per image (lower than one for Haar descriptor). We can also notice that, for both descriptors, the average detection latency is now more than a second. We associate this to false positives damaging posterior good detections. Only Haar presents a MCT compatible with real time constraints

Table 3. Impact of Paris morphology on overall performance results. N1 classifiers are used for both for LBP and Haar features, as well as spatio-temporal coherence.

Method	MNFP	Prec	Rec	F1	RT
0-Is (sessile,11 polyps)					
LBPN1	1.3	23.93%	40.84%	30.18%	40.6 [1.6 sec]
HaarN1	0.6	38.01%	41.32%	39.59%	22.3 [0.9 sec]
Aggregation	1.2	27.93%	48.18%	35.36%	21 [0.8 sec]
0-Ip (peduncular,3 polyps)					
LBPN1	1.0	31.4%	51.10%	38.90%	89.0 [3.6 sec]
HaarN1	0.5	50.46%	57.50%	53.75%	4.0 [0.1 sec]
Aggregation	1.1	40.28%	64.73%	49.66%	4.0 [0.1 sec]
0-IIa (flat, 4 polyps)					
LBPN1	1.1	34.62%	59.35%	43.73%	18.0 [0.7 sec]
HaarN1	0.6	35.14%	37.08%	36.08%	58.5 [2.3 sec]
Aggregation	0.8	32.32%	58.10%	41.54%	7.0 [0.3 sec]

(36 ms). Considering the overall positive impact of spatio temporal coherence, in the following it will be applied for all experiments.

Though clearly more specific to the reference methodology used, Table 2 shows the benefit of the strengthening strategy for both descriptors. The overall performance is improved though, for the case of LBP, the mean computation time remains incompatible with a clinical use, and the detection latency is not far from 2 s for $LBPN2$ classifier. Haar descriptors definitely appear here more compatible with a daily routine use since for $HaarN1$ the mean latency is only of 1.1 s but with 14 videos (on the overall 18) presenting with an average RT lower than 0.4 s; the mean computation time is only of 21 ms with a max value of only 25 ms for video 14 and, finally, the overall performance levels obtained are the best from all the experiments presented in this paper in terms of trade-off between true and false alarms.

One of the reasons of studying the use of different type of features was to observe whether the *combination of several feature types* could lead to an overall performance improvement. Our experiments yield an interesting result: the combination of LBP and Haar classifiers leads to a significant increase of the TP detection rate since the Recall reaches its highest value considering the all set of experiments achieved in this section. Results indicate that LBP and Haar can detect different kind of polyp (RoIs) in a complementary way. Nevertheless, from a clinical applicability perspective, even if the mean RT is only of 0.7 s when combining both classifiers, as expected, the mean processing time per frame is constrained by LBP classifier performance which is of an average value of more than 185 ms. Finally, we can observe in Table 3 how the combination of feature descriptors help to improve recall scores and to reduce computation time regardless polyp morphology.

The first conclusion that we can extract from the analysis of the results presented is that our proposed adaptation strategy does improve the performance of still-frame based methods when dealing with video analysis. The use of spatio-temporal coherence leads to a reduction in the number of false positive alarms whereas the combination of different types of features lead to an increase in the number of polyp frames correctly detected. It is important to mention that some of these improvements come at the cost of losing real-time capabilities and efforts should be made to improve the computational cost of some of the proposed improvements (such as the combination of LBP and Haar features).

5 Discussion

5.1 Impact of Adaptation Strategy on Method's Performance

With respect of the specific feature descriptor used, we observed better performance related to the use of Haar features. We associate this to the fact that in video sequences, differences in texture between mucosa and the polyp become less relevant and, in this case, the presence of strong boundaries delimiting the different structures such as polyps in the image may appear more useful than texture analysis. Nevertheless, it has to be taken into account LBP's offers best performance for the case of flat polyps, which are those recurrently mentioned by clinicians as one of the main causes of polyp miss-rate. If the decision on the descriptor to use depends on real time constraints, Haar is the way to go but, as Fig. 5(a–d) shows, the combination of both descriptors might increase overall performance.

With respect to spatio-temporal coherence module, its inclusion has led to a reduction in the number of false alarms but it has also lead to a decrease in performance scores on Recall or RT. We associate this decrease to isolated correct detections not kept through consecutive frames therefore leading to miss the polyp in the whole subsequence of frames. In this case efforts should be made to clearly identify the polyp target to be tracked in order to only mitigate false alarms and not those correct ones. Consequently, efforts should be put on

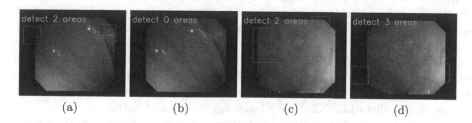

| (a)   (b)   (c)   (d) |

Fig. 5. Differences in performance associated to the specific feature descriptor used: (a, c) show the output of Haar descriptor whereas (b, d) show the output achieved using LBP as descriptor.

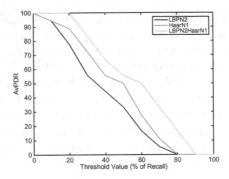

Fig. 6. Evolution of the AvPDR metric with respect to the threshold value applied to the Recall on each video.

identifying and tackling appropriately the source of those false alarms which might involve, as some authors propose [4], considering the impact of other elements of the endoluminal scene.

5.2 Frame-Based Analysis vs. Clinical Applicability

We have presented in Sect. 3 two sets of metrics to represent the performance of a given method. It is clear that clinicians will be mainly interested on whether the computational system is able to detect the polyp once it appears in the image. As the polyp is detected, their attention will deviate to other areas in the image. Considering this, a good performing method could be one that only detects the polyp in one frame being this frame the first in which the polyp appears in the sequence. As this kind of system does not warrantee good performance under exploratory conditions, frame-based and clinical applicability metrics should be combined to represent actual method performance.

To solve this, we propose to combine the most clinically relevant metric (PDR) with Recall into a new metric representing both whether the method is able to detect the polyp and that this detection occurs in a relevant number of frames. We define the Average Polyp Detection Rate (AvPDR) to checks whether a method is able to detect the polyp in a set of sequences with respect to a minimum value for Recall. We calculate AvPDR in the following way: for each video we set individual (IndPDR) score to 1 if Recall score for the particular video surpasses Rec_{thres} value. Final AvPDR score for the whole dataset will be calculated as the mean of individual InDPRs. To illustrate this, Fig. 6 shows the evolution of the AvPDR for different values of the Recall and for the three last computed classifiers LBPN2, HaarN1 and aggregation of both.

As it can be seen, the AvPDR brings very interesting insights on the capacity of a given method to detect the polyp with a given minimum Recall. In our case, the aggregation of LBPN2 and HaarN1 classifiers makes possible to systematically detect the polyp in all videos with a minimum Recall of 20%.

5.3 Analysis of Methods' Performance in the Context of the State-of-the-Art

As mentioned in Sect. 1, there are many available polyp detection methods in the literature, some of them already showing quite good performance as it can be observed in [5]. The main objective of our work was not to develop the best polyp detection method but to show how still frame-based methodologies databases could still be valid for full sequences analysis.

Due to the lack of publicly available annotated video databases, we can only compare global performance scores of different methods even if they have not been tested under the same conditions. In this sense, our approach obtains similar performances in PDR and Reaction time than those achieved by the best methods presented in [5]. As mentioned before, we are not worried here about frame-based performance (though it has to be improved for sure) but on whether the system can be of actual clinical use hence the focus on real time performance. We also believe that, once public video databases become more available, methods performance (especially machine learning ones) will benefit from being trained on them as they will cover a wide variety of polyp appearances.

Finally and to assess actual clinical applicability of a given method on the exploration room, we believe efforts should also be made on incorporating full realistic interventions as part of the databases in a way such once the polyp is found the clinician progresses through the colon without the need of observing the polyp in different views, typical from still frame database creation protocols,

6 Conclusions

We have presented in this paper a study on how to adapt still frame based polyp detection methodologies to full sequences analysis. Our adaptation strategy involves the addition of a spatio-temporal coherence module and the combination of feature descriptors. We have tested the impact (in performance and computational efficiency) of this adaptation strategy implementing them over an already existing real time polyp detection method trained on still frame based databases. We validate the complete methodology over a newly published video database of 18 sequences using a set of clinical and technical performance metrics.

The main conclusion extracted from this study is that the addition of a spatio-temporal coherence module and the combination of feature descriptors lead to an overall improvement on method performance over full sequences; once these modules are applied over the reference method, the proposed methodology is able to detect all different polyps in at least one frame in the sequence.

It has to be noted that the best performing configuration is not ready for clinical use due to not meeting real time constraints; efforts should be made to increase the computational efficiency of the different modules proposed. Apart from this, we also foresee the following areas of improvement: (i) add an image preprocessing stage to mitigate the impact of other elements of the endoluminal scene (which can impact when the first correct detection occurs), (ii) incorporate computationally efficient camera motion tracking methods to improve spatio-temporal coherence and (iii) study the possibility of incorporating additional feature descriptors to improve overall performance. Moreover, our method should be trained over video sequences in order to capture better the great variability of polyp appearance within a same sequence.

Acknowledgements. The authors acknowledge the support of the following agencies for research funding: Spanish government through funded project iVENDIS (DPI2015-65286-R), SATT IdFInnov (France) through the Project Smart Videocolonoscopy under Grant 186, Catalan government through SGR projects 2014-SGR-1470 and 2014-SGR-135, CERCA Programme/Generalitat de Catalunya and FSEED.

References

1. ACS2016: Key statistics for colorectal cancer. online (2016)
2. Angermann, Q., Histace, A., Romain, O.: Active learning for real time detection of polyps in videocolonoscopy. Procedia Comput. Sci. **90**, 182–187 (2016)
3. Bernal, J., Histace, A.: Gastrointestinal Image Analysis (GIANA) sub-challenge. online (2017)
4. Bernal, J., Sánchez, F.J., Fernández-Esparrach, G., et al.: Wm-dova maps for accurate polyp highlighting in colonoscopy: validation vs. saliency maps from physicians. Comput. Med. Imaging Graph. **43**, 99–111 (2015)
5. Bernal, J., Tajbakhsh, N., et al.: Comparative validation of polyp detection methods in video colonoscopy: Results from the MICCAI 2015 endoscopic vision challenge. IEEE Trans. Med. Imaging **36**(6), 1231–1249 (2017). doi:10.1109/TMI.2017.2664042
6. Bruno, M.: Magnification endoscopy, high resolution endoscopy, and chromoscopy; towards a better optical diagnosis. Gut **52**(suppl. 4), iv7–iv11 (2003)
7. Coriat, R., Chryssostalis, A., Zeitoun, J., et al.: Computed virtual chromoendoscopy system (FICE): a new tool for upper endoscopy? Gastroentérologie clinique et biologique **32**(4), 363–369 (2008)
8. Gross, S., Stehle, T., Behrens, A., et al.: A comparison of blood vessel features and local binary patterns for colorectal polyp classification. In: SPIE Medical Imaging, p. 72,602Q. International Society for Optics and Photonics (2009)
9. Inoue, H., Kashida, H., Kudo, et al.: The paris endoscopic classification of superficial neoplastic lesions: esophagus, stomach, and colon: November 30 to december 1, 2002. Gastrointest Endosc **58**(6 Suppl.), S3–S43 (2003)
10. Leufkens, A., van Oijen, M., Vleggaar, F., Siersema, P.: Factors influencing the miss rate of polyps in a back-to-back colonoscopy study. Endoscopy **44**(05), 470–475 (2012)
11. Lienhart, R., Maydt, J.: An extended set of haar-like features for rapid object detection. In: Proceedings of the 2002 International Conference on Image Processing, vol. 1, p. I-900. IEEE (2002)
12. Machida, H., Sano, Y., Hamamoto, Y., et al.: Narrow-band imaging in the diagnosis of colorectal mucosal lesions: a pilot study. Endoscopy **36**(12), 1094–1098 (2004)
13. Park, S.Y., Sargent, D.: Colonoscopic polyp detection using convolutional neural networks. In: SPIE Medical Imaging, pp. 978, 528–978, 528. International Society for Optics and Photonics (2016)

14. Tajbakhsh, N., Gurudu, S.R., Liang, J.: Automatic polyp detection in colonoscopy videos using an ensemble of convolutional neural networks. In: 2015 IEEE 12th International Symposium on Biomedical Imaging (ISBI), pp. 79–83. IEEE (2015)
15. Wang, Y., Tavanapong, W., Wong, J., et al.: Polyp-alert: Near real-time feedback during colonoscopy. Comput. Methods Programs Biomed. **120**(3), 164–179 (2015)
16. Wang, Z., Song, Y., Zhang, C.: Efficient active learning with boosting. In: Proceedings of the SIAM International Conference on Data Mining Society for Industrial and Applied Mathematics, pp. 1232–1243. Society for Industrial and Applied Mathematics (2009)

Progressive Hand-Eye Calibration
for Laparoscopic Surgery Navigation

Jinliang Shao[1,2], Huoling Luo[1,3], Deqiang Xiao[1,3], Qingmao Hu[1,3],
and Fucang Jia[1,3(✉)]

[1] Shenzhen Institutes of Advanced Technology,
Chinese Academy of Sciences, Shenzhen 518055, China
fc.jia@siat.ac.cn
[2] Sino-Dutch Biomedical and Information Engineering School,
Northeastern University, Shenyang 110819, China
[3] Shenzhen College of Advanced Technology,
University of Chinese Academy of Sciences, Shenzhen 518055, China

Abstract. In this paper, we presented a progressive strategy based on an invariant point to accomplish hand-eye calibration for laparoscopic surgery navigation. An invariant dot was imaged by a stereo laparoscopy, the 2D image coordinate of the invariant dot was calculated by the blob detection algorithm, and mapped into the 3D coordinate system by the triangulation. In the meanwhile, reflective passive markers (RPM) fixed on the distal end of a stereo laparoscope was located by an optical tracking system. The Levenberg-Marquardt (LM) algorithm was used to iteratively estimate the hand-eye transformation based on the dot image coordinates and RPM's poses. One pair of dot image coordinate and RPM's pose were acquired in each iteration procedure, and were added into their accumulated data buffer as the input of LM optimization. The calibration error was calculated as well for each iteration. To evaluate accuracy of the proposed method, laboratory experiments were conducted by computing two errors, including forward error and backward error. The results show that the minimal forward error of 1.32 mm and backward error of 0.86 pixels were obtained at the 8th iteration. In conclusion, the high calibration accuracy can be achieved with a few progressive iterations by our method. Additionally, the proposed approach provided a way for operators to monitor the procedure so that the calibration process can be stopped when the procedure feedbacks an acceptable accuracy.

Keywords: Hand-eye calibration · Laparoscopic surgery navigation · Progressive calibration · Invariant point

1 Introduction

Laparoscopic surgery is a popular clinical procedure because of its minimal invasiveness and shorter postoperative hospital stays relative to open surgery. However, this procedure is always limited by restricted field of view and lack of tactile feedback.

J. Shao and H. Luo are contributed equally.

© Springer International Publishing AG 2017
M.J. Cardoso et al. (Eds.): CARE/CLIP 2017, LNCS 10550, pp. 42–49, 2017.
DOI: 10.1007/978-3-319-67543-5_4

To overcome these limitations, image-guided surgery system [1] and surgical robotic [2] have been developed. Hand-eye calibration is a well-known term in robotics literature; for laparoscopic surgery navigation, "hand" denotes the reflective passive markers (RPM) attached to the laparoscope, and "eye" denotes the laparoscopic camera. Hand-eye calibration determines the position and orientation of the laparoscopic camera relative to the (RPM), is an important procedure for implementing a navigation system for laparoscopic surgery.

The hand-eye calibration can be formulated as a linear system of equations as:

$$\mathbf{AX} = \mathbf{XB} \tag{1}$$

where $\mathbf{A}$ denotes the relative motion of laparoscopic camera, $\mathbf{B}$ is the motion of the RPM, and $\mathbf{X}$ represents the hand-eye transformation. Tsai and Lenz [3] have proven that at least two motions are required to solve Eq. (1).

Many methods have been proposed to estimate the hand-eye transformation. It can be decomposed into a rotation matrix and a translation vector. The most commonly used method was realized by computing the rotation and the translation separately [4], while the rotation and the translation can also be jointly estimated [5]. Horaud et al. [6] proved that the camera intrinsic calibration is not independent from hand-eye calibration. Malm and Heyden [7] investigated a joint solution for a camera intrinsic calibration and hand-eye calibration using an unfixed planar calibration object for robot vision. Malti et al. [8] proposed a similar hand-eye calibration approach, they estimated the optimal camera parameters as well as hand-eye transformation based on the minimal number of the calibration object images.

Although hand-eye calibration has been well-studied within robotic field, it is challenging to transfer these methods from robotic literature into laparoscopic surgery directly. Because different situations existed in laparoscopic surgery, the proposed method is required to be compatible with sterility constrains and not to interrupt the surgical workflow. Recently, Thompson et al. [9] proposed a novel calibration method for laparoscopic surgery navigation. In their work, an invariant cross-hair point was imaged by a stereo laparoscope with different views; positions of the invariant point were automatically calculated from laparoscopic images, and the Levenberg-Marquardt (LM) optimizer was used to estimate an optimal hand-eye transformation based on extracted invariant points and poses of RPM. However, the accuracy of their method would be compromised with inaccurate cross-hair detection or outlier data input.

Inspired by the work of Thompson et al. [9], we proposed a progressive strategy based on an invariant point for hand-eye calibration. In this strategy, the hand-eye transform of the i-th iteration was initialized with the results of i-1 iteration, and updated based on the accumulation data buffer of the i-th iteration. Different from the invariant point used in Thompson's work, a fixed small dot acting as the invariant point was applied in our method. To evaluate accuracy of the proposed method, two errors were calculated at each iteration. With the iterative evaluation, the operator can set a desired error prior to calibration and terminates the hand-eye calibration when the procedure gives an acceptable value.

2 Methods

2.1 Hardware

The hardware used in this study is shown in Fig. 1. A Polaris Spectra optical tracking system (NDI, Waterloo, Ontario, Canada) was employed to record the pose of RPM. Because the clinical stereo laparoscope is not available, two Ultra Mini CMOS Color Cameras (MISUMI) were assembled to make a stereo laparoscope (Fig. 1A), its spatial resolution is 640 × 480 and baseline is 6 cm. The RPM is fixed on the distal end of the stereo laparoscope. To improve the accuracy of the invariant point detection, we did not use the cross-hair as an invariant point, any sterile paper marked with one dot can be used as a calibration object in our work. To guarantee the accuracy of invariant point extraction, the diameter of the dot was set as 1 mm.

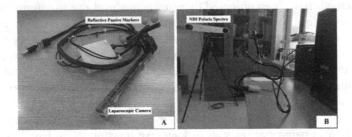

Fig. 1. (A) Custom-made stereo laparoscope and (B) hand-eye calibration theatre setting.

2.2 Progressive Hand-Eye Calibration

The stereo laparoscopic camera was calibrated prior to hand-eye calibration. To obtain the camera intrinsic and extrinsic parameters, the widely used checkboard method [10] from OpenCV was applied directly. Because the focal length is fixed in custom-made laparoscope, camera calibration can be performed prior to the clinical procedure and saved to a file for the usage at any time. During the procedure of hand-eye calibration, the laparoscope camera was kept above the dot calibration object, and the RPM was tracked by the optical positional tracker at the same time. We rotated the laparoscope within a cone to acquire laparoscopic images of the invariant point (Fig. 2); in this cone, the vertex is roughly located at the dot, and the rotation angle is about 60°.

We proposed a strategy that laparoscopic images of the calibration object were iteratively acquired and processed to get an optimal hand-eye transformation. Figure 3 shows the workflow of the proposed method. After capturing the left/right images of the variant dot, both images were converted into grayscale format and smoothed, the blob detection algorithm was applied to detect 2D image coordinates of the dot centroid. Based on previously determined camera intrinsic and extrinsic parameters, the 3D coordinate of the dot centroid in the left camera coordinate system was computed by triangulation. The 3D coordinate is defined as X_{L_i}, where i denotes the number of iterations. Meanwhile, the optical position tracking system captured the pose of RPM, $^{tracker}T_{hand\_i}$, at the same time.

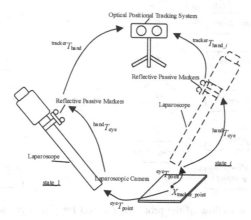

Fig. 2. Rotate the laparoscope within a cone, its vertex is roughly located at the dot, and its angle is about 60°.

Considering that the ith iteration, the coordinate of the invariant point defined in the left camera space, X_{L_i}, can be transformed to the optical tracker coordinate system (see the relationship of transformations as shown in Fig. 2), X_{world_i}, according to the following equation,

$$X_{world\_i} = {}^{tracker}T_{hand\_i} \times {}^{hand}T_{eye} \times X_{L\_i} \qquad (2)$$

Meanwhile, we denote the 3D coordinate of invariant point defined in optical tracker system space as $X_{tracker\_point} = (x_t, y_t, z_t)$. Therefore, there are two vectors, X_{world_i} and $X_{tracker\_point}$, representing coordinates for the same invariant point. Theoretically, these two vectors should be identical or the residual error E between them is as small as possible,

$$E_j = X_{world\_i,j} - X_{tracker\_point\_j} \qquad (3)$$

where j represents the x, y, z components of $X_{tracker\_point}$.

The hand-eye transformation can be represented as a matrix, $\begin{bmatrix} R & t \\ \vec{0} & 1 \end{bmatrix}$, where R denotes a rotation with three components, and t is a translation which is also can be divided into three scalars. Thus, there is a total of nine parameters, including R, t, and three components of $X_{tracker\_point}$ to be optimized. Levenberg-Marquardt optimizer algorithm was employed to optimize the unknown parameters based on Eq. (3), which is initialized with $X_{tracker\_point} = (0, 0, 0)$ and an identity matrix of ${}^{hand}T_{eye}$.

A strategy that progressively adding new frames of the invariant dot into the workflow to optimize the obtained hand-eye transform was used. We acquired one frame data of the variant dot from the laparoscopic space and the tracking system space, respectively. After adding the newly acquired data into the data buffer obtained before, a new accumulated data buffer was set as the input for LM algorithm to re-optimize the hand-eye transform.

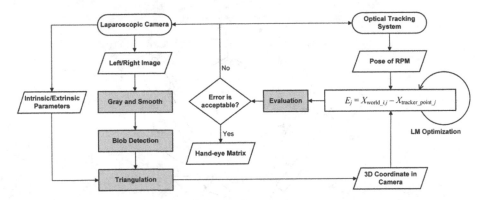

Fig. 3. The workflow of the proposed method for hand-eye calibration.

The calibration error was evaluated at each iteration. Before the calibration, we located the invariant dot in the optical tracking system with a tracking probe from the Polaris Spectra system, then the 3D coordinate of the invariant dot, $X_{\text{tracker\_point}}$, was obtained. Based on the calculated hand-eye transform, the 3D coordinate of the invariant dot in the optical tracking system can be mapped into the 2D image coordinate system according to the following equation,

$$X_{\text{L\_project\_}i} = {}^{\text{hand}}T_{\text{eye}}^{-1} \times {}^{\text{tracker}}T_{\text{hand\_}i}^{-1} \times X_{\text{tracker\_point}} \tag{4}$$

where $X_{\text{L\_project\_}i}$ denotes the mapped 2D image coordinate; the calibration error is evaluated as the distance (in pixel) between the mapped invariant dot and the corresponding ground truth in the laparoscopic image. We evaluated the calibration error iteratively. The iteration terminates once the error meets the input tolerance, otherwise; hand-eye calibration program will progressively collect the new frames to perform the next iteration until the error is acceptable.

3 Experiments

The ground truth data were acquired before calibration to evaluate accuracy of the proposed method. Through the blob detection, the 2D image coordinate of the variant dot, $X_{\text{L\_base}}$, was computed from laparoscopic images. At the same time, a probe from Polaris Spectra system was used to locate the position of invariant dot in the tracker coordinate system, $X_{\text{tracker\_base}}$. The $X_{\text{L\_base}}$ and $X_{\text{tracker\_base}}$ were used as the ground truth data for the method evaluation. The proposed hand-eye calibration approach was implemented based on an open-source toolkit of MITK [11] as shown in Fig. 4.

The forward and backward errors were calculated to assess the calibration accuracy. Based on the obtained hand-eye transform after each iteration, a 2D image coordinate of the variant dot $X_{\text{L\_test}}$, can be mapped into the optical tracker coordinate system to get a 3D coordinate $X_{\text{tracker\_test}}$, by applying Eq. (2). The forward error is defined as the distance (in mm) between $X_{\text{tracker\_test}}$ and the ground truth $X_{\text{tracker\_base}}$, on the contrary,

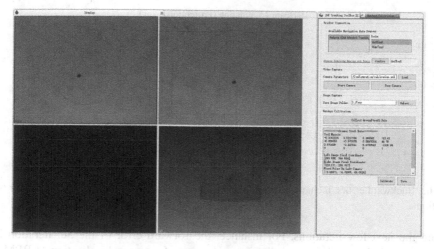

Fig. 4. The graphic user interface of the hand-eye calibration implemented using MITK.

by applying Eq. (4), the point coordinate estimated from LM optimization, denoted as $X_{tracker\_estimated}$, can be mapped into 2D laparoscopic image coordinate system. The backward error is defined as the distance (in pixel) between mapped 2D coordinate, donated as $X_{L\_estimated}$, and the corresponding ground truth X_{L_base}.

4 Results

A total of 70 frames data were collected to evaluate calibration accuracy. The forward and backward errors are depicted in Figs. 5 and 6, respectively.

The accuracy of the proposed method can be guaranteed when the outlier data was collected, because the procedure can be reinitialized with a reasonable value from a previous iteration without outlier data, and the error would fall into an acceptable range

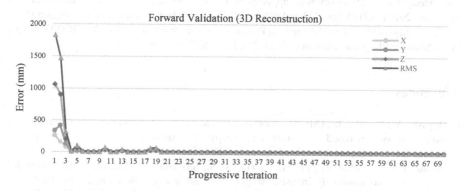

Fig. 5. Forward errors, including the total error and its three components were calculated for 60 iterations.

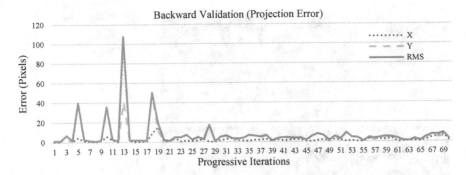

Fig. 6. Backward errors, including the total error and its two components were calculated for 60 iterations.

during the next few iterations. For instance, the forward error of the 5th iteration is 41.95 mm. Obviously, it is an outlier input because of a wrong localization of RPM's pose, while the error can be decreased into a reasonable range after several iterations. At the same iteration, the projected error is 39.77 pixels, but the error is also decreased during the following iterations. The minimum errors were obtained at the 8th iteration with forward error of 1.32 mm and the backward error of 0.86 pixels, respectively.

5   Conclusion

In this paper, we presented a progressive strategy based on an invariant dot to accomplish the hand-eye calibration for laparoscopic surgery navigation. The calibration accuracy was evaluated by forward and backward errors in the laboratory experiments. The results show that the high calibration accuracy can be obtained with a few progressive iterations. In addition, the proposed method provided a way for operators to monitor the calibration procedure; they can stop the calibration when the procedure feedbacks an acceptable accuracy.

Acknowledgments. This work was supported by the national key research & development program (Nos. 2016YFC0106500/502 and SQ2017ZY040217/03), the NSFC Union program (Nos. U1401254 and U1613221), the Guangdong Provincial Scientific Program (No. 2015B020214005), and the Shenzhen Key Basic Science Grant (No. JCYJ20170413162213765).

References

1. Hayashi, Y., Misawa, K., Oda, M., Hawkes, D.J., Mori, K.: Clinical application of a surgical navigation system based on virtual laparoscopy in laparoscopic gastrectomy for gastric cancer. Int. J. Comput. Assist. Radiol. Surg. **11**(5), 827–836 (2016)
2. Pachtrachai, K., Allan, M., Pawar, V., Hailes, S., Stoyanov, D.: Hand-eye calibration for robotic assisted minimally invasive surgery without a calibration object. In: IEEE/RSJ International Conference on Intelligent Robots and Systems (IROS), pp. 2485–2491, October 2016

3. Tsai, R.Y., Lenz, R.K.: Real time versatile robotics hand/eye calibration using 3D machine vision. In: IEEE Transactions on Robotics and Automation, pp. 554–561, April 1988
4. Tsai, R.Y., Lenz, R.K.: A new technique for fully autonomous and efficient 3D robotics hand/eye calibration. IEEE Trans. Robot. Autom. **5**(3), 345–358 (1989)
5. Daniilidis, K.: Hand-eye calibration using dual quaternions. Int. J. Robot. Res. **18**(3), 286–298 (1999)
6. Horaud, R., Dornaika, F.: Hand-eye calibration. Int. J. Robot. Res. **14**(3), 195–210 (1995)
7. Malm, H., Heyden, A.: Simplified intrinsic camera calibration and hand-eye calibration for robot vision. In: IEEE/RSJ International Conference on Intelligent Robots and Systems (IROS), pp. 1037–1043, October 2003
8. Malti, A., Barreto, J.P.: Hand–eye and radial distortion calibration for rigid endoscopes. Int. J. Med. Robot. Comput. Assist. Surg. **9**(4), 441–454 (2013)
9. Thompson, S., Stoyanov, D., Schneider, C., Gurusamy, K., Ourselin, S., Davidson, B., Hawkes, D., Clarkson, M.J.: Hand–eye calibration for rigid laparoscopes using an invariant point. Int. J. Comput. Assist. Radiol. Surg. **11**(6), 1071–1080 (2016)
10. Zhang, Z.: A flexible new technique for camera calibration. IEEE Trans. Pattern Anal. Mach. Intell. **22**(11), 1330–1334 (2000)
11. Nolden, M., Zelzer, S., Seitel, A., et al.: The medical imaging interaction toolkit: challenges and advances. Int. J. Comput. Assist. Radiol. Surg. **8**(4), 607–620 (2013)

Learning Camera Pose from Optical Colonoscopy Frames Through Deep Convolutional Neural Network (CNN)

Mohammad Ali Armin[1,2(✉)], Nick Barnes[1,4], Jose Alvarez[1],
Hongdong Li[4], Florian Grimpen[3], and Olivier Salvado[2]

[1] CSIRO (Data61), Canberra, Australia
m.a.armin@gmail.com, Nick.Barnes@data61.csiro.au,
Olivier.Salvado@csiro.au
[2] Biomedical Informatics Group, Brisbane, Australia
[3] Department of Gastroenterology and Hepatology,
Royal Brisbane and Women's Hospital, Brisbane, Australia
[4] College of Engineering and Computer Science (ANU),
Canberra, Australia

Abstract. Optical colonoscopy is performed by insertion of a long flexible colonoscope into the colon. Estimating the position of the colonoscope tip with respect to the colon surface is important as it would help localization of cancerous polyps for subsequent surgery and facilitate navigation. Knowing camera pose is also essential for 3D automatic scene reconstruction, which could support clinicians inspecting the whole colon surface thereby reducing missed polyps. This paper presents a method to estimate the pose of the colonoscope camera with six degrees of freedom (DoF) using deep convolutional neural network (CNN). Because obtaining a ground truth to train the CNN for camera pose from actual colonoscopy videos is extremely challenging, we trained the CNN using realistic synthetic videos generated with a colonoscopy simulator, which could generate the exact camera pose parameters. We validated the trained CNN on unseen simulated video datasets and on actual colonoscopy videos from 10 patients. Our results showed that the colonoscopy camera pose could be estimated with higher accuracy and speed than feature based computer vision methods such as the classical structure from motion (SfM) pipeline. This paper demonstrates that transfer learning from surgical simulation to actual endoscopic based surgery is a possible approach for deep learning technologies.

Keywords: Optical colonoscopy · Convolutional neural network (CNN) · Camera pose

---

Electronic supplementary material The online version of this chapter (doi:10.1007/978-3-319-67543-5_5) contains supplementary material, which is available to authorized users.

M.J. Cardoso et al. (Eds.): CARE/CLIP 2017, LNCS 10550, pp. 50–59, 2017.
DOI: 10.1007/978-3-319-67543-5_5

1 Introduction

Colorectal cancer is ranked as the type of cancer that is third most likely to claim people's lives in Australia, and the fourth worldwide [1, 2]. Optical colonoscopy has been known as the gold standard method for detecting and removing colonic polyps, the precursor of bowel cancer [3].

Estimating the colonoscope position with high accuracy is important as it can determine the location of detected polyps, especially when there is a need for subsequent surgery for removing cancerous polyps [4]. Despite the work that has been done in estimating the colonoscope position (camera pose) from optical colonoscopy [5, 6], accurately localizing the position of colonoscope with respect to the colon's surface remains a critical issue.

Conventional methods to estimate camera motion from an endoscopy procedure such as optical flow [5–7] or hybrid methods [8, 9] are time consuming, sensitive to feature matching, require an offline camera or sensor calibration and resulted in a drift in camera pose estimation. Here, we develop a method based on deep convolutional neural network (CNN) to estimate relative camera pose between two consecutive frames, which is independent to traditional feature detection and tracking, and reduces the camera drift.

In recent years, convolutional neural networks have been widely used in various computer vision fields. Although they were initially designed for classification purposes [10], the recent CNNs with advanced architectures have shown significant results in problems including object recognition [11], optical flow estimation [12], and dense feature matching [13] by means of simulated or actual data. Using artificial neural networks (ANN), Bell et al. [14] estimated the camera pose of teleoperated flexible endoscopes by training ANNs with optical flow magnitude and angle when the endoscope was moved by a robotic hand inside a plastic colon phantom. Recently, Kendall et al. [15] regressed the camera pose from a single RGB image by training a CNN with camera pose which was estimated offline by a structure from motion algorithm as ground truth. The main challenge then was lack of ground truth for scenes which had not enough features to track to estimate ground truth through SfM. Since annotating real images is difficult and expensive, application of synthetic data has boosted its popularity as an alternative to train networks [16, 17].

In this paper, we aim to estimate camera pose from actual optical colonoscopy video frames. To achieve this, rather than using SfM [15] to generate a ground truth, we trained a CNN by simulated colonoscopy frames for which the camera poses were available from the simulator as ground truth. The camera pose for actual colonoscopy frames was then regressed when the actual colonoscopy frames were passed to the network. The results obtained from the CNN were compared to a feature based algorithm which is explained in [18]. In addition, the performance of different networks architecture and input data (optical flow) were investigated. A diagram of our method is demonstrated in Fig. 1 and described in the following sections.

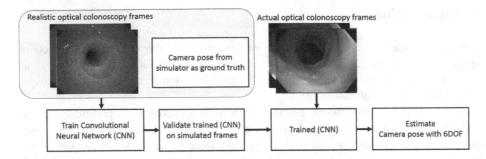

Fig. 1. Main processing steps of our proposed method

2 Method

We presented two approaches, we trained the CNN by optical flow patterns between consecutive frames, by or alternatively directly by consecutive frames. The camera pose parameters inferred from the CNN were compared to a structure from motion (SfM) algorithm [18]. First we briefly describe the preprocessing including frame preparation for training CNNs with frames, SIFT flow [19] estimation for training with motion field, and SfM as a camera pose estimation method, before explaining the proposed CNN's model architecture and training details.

2.1 Pre-processing and SfM

Frames were prepared through the following steps; (i) frames were converted to grayscale, (ii) the black corners were removed as they had no information (iii) frames were resized to train modified AlexNet and GoogLeNet. The size of input data (*height* × *width* × *number of frames*) for AlexNet and GoogLeNet were (227 × 227 × 2), (224 × 224 × 2) respectively. To estimate the optical flow pattern, the SIFT flow algorithm [19] was utilized to extract and match features between two consecutive grayscale frames. The final input data had the size of (227 × 227 × 2), and included motion field in u and v direction.

2.2 Model for Estimating Camera Pose

In this section, we describe the CNN models that estimate the camera pose parameters. The input to our models are either: the two consecutive grayscale frames; or optical flow pattern between consecutive frames. The outputs are relative camera translations and rotations with respect to the colon surface with six degrees of freedom (DoF).

Learning camera translation and rotation. Camera rotation and translation parameters were regressed by training the CNN to minimize the following objective function:

$$Loss = \beta \cdot \left\| R_{target} - R_{predicted} \right\|^2 + \left\| T_{target} - T_{predicted} \right\|^2$$

Where β is the weight factor for our dataset is one, (R_{target}, T_{target}) are camera rotation (degree) and translation (mm) which are available from the simulator as ground truth, and $(R_{predicetd}, T_{predicetd})$ are camera pose parameters predicted by the CNN. The camera translation is normalized to unit vector and is unit less. In our experiments, the camera rotation is represented in Eulerian angle (α, ψ, γ). Applying Euclidian distance on Euler angle may result in more than one set of values which can yield the same angle representation. According to [21], this can be prevented under the following conditions on the Euler angles: $\alpha, \gamma \in [-\pi, \pi)$; $\psi \in [-\pi/2, \pi/2)$, and therefore L2 on rotation is a metric on SO(3) [21]. In our dataset the maximum of relative rotation is below the mentioned range in [21].

Network architecture. The base of the architecture of our CNN is the state-of-the-art GoogLeNet for the direct image pair. We also modified AlexNet for the optical flow approach to compare the results. These networks were originally designed for image classification. We applied the following changes on both GoogLeNet and AlexNet to regress the camera parameters; (i) considering the input data to the network, which are motion features (u,v) in two dimensions or two consecutive frames in grayscale, the first convolutional layer filter (filter size; input channel; number of filters) was modified to (11;2;96) for AlexNet and (7;2;4) for GoogelNet, allowing networks to operate in two dimensions; and (ii) the Softmax classifier was replaced by two fully connected

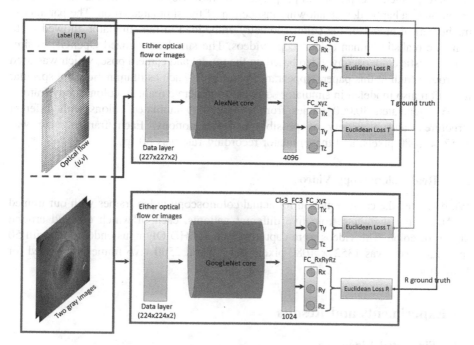

Fig. 2. The general architecture of our CNNs to predict camera pose parameters, the first layer is modified to accept two gray images or optical flow, and the classification layer was replaced by Euclidean loss to optimize predicted rotation and translation by network. Note that we trained AlexNet with both optical flow and image for comparison purposes.

layers, each with three outputs to estimate relative camera rotation and translation. The outputs of last layers then passed to a Euclidean loss function to regress the camera pose. The schematic of our networks are shown in Fig. 2.

Training details and transfer learning. The Matconvnet toolbox [22] was used for the implementation of our CNN model. We trained our network using stochastic gradient descent on our dataset which included 30,000 grayscale frames and their optical flow patterns. The batch size and iteration were 580 and 2500 respectively. To prevent any bias, input data were shuffled and randomly chosen for each batch. Since the pre-trained networks were used for our experiments, the learning rate was initialized to be 10^{-4}, and every 1000 epochs it was reduced by 0.1, and the momentum was set to 0.9. We used multi-GPU (Nvidia) for training to accelerate the training computational speed. The trained networks by simulated data then were used to predict camera pose from actual colonoscopy videos.

3   Dataset

3.1   Simulated Video

The simulated colonoscopy video frames were generated by the CSIRO colonoscopy simulator, which is explained in [23]. The simulator uses a 3D analytical model of the colon, with a haptic device allowing inspection of the simulated colon. The parametric mathematical model of the colon geometry embedded in the simulator allowed us to generate realistic human colonoscopy videos. The simulator utilized OpenGL to simulate realistic colonoscopy video based on the model and camera pose, which was used as ground truth in this paper. Appearance parameters such as illumination and specular reflection also modeled in simulator software to generate realistic colonoscopy frames.

We generated 30,000 frames from 15 different simulated colons with different structures, and a variety of possible camera motions. Each frame's size was 1352×1080 pixels, and the simulator recording rate was 30 fps.

3.2   Real Colonoscopy Video

We predicted the camera motion for actual colonoscopy video frames with our trained CNN on five segments from five different patients, each of which covered around 20 cm of colon. The videos were captured by a 190HD Olympus endoscope, with 50 fps (frame size was 1352×1080 pixels). In general 2500 vivo frames were used for validation.

4   Experiments and Results

4.1   Simulated Video

The networks were trained with 80% of data (chosen from different videos), which were shuffled to prevent bias in the training phase. The trained networks with optical

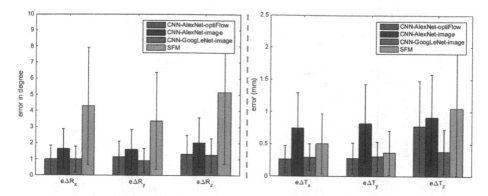

Fig. 3. The root mean square error (RMS) and standard deviation (STD) between ground truth and the camera rotations and translations estimated by SfM, modified AlexNet trained by optical flow and grayscale frames, and modified GoogLeNet trained by grayscale frames.

flow pattern and two consecutive grayscale frames were tested on the remaining data. In our study to demonstrate the performance of CNNs in comparison to a feature based algorithm; we estimated motion features between consecutive frames, removed uninformative frames [20] and computed camera translation and rotation with respect to the colon surface [18]. The results including the root mean square error (RMS) and standard deviation (STD) from the ground truth for both CNNs and SfM are shown in Fig. 3. The results indicate the higher performance of modified GoogLeNet trained by grayscale frames in comparison to other methods.

To investigate the ability of the trained networks in generalizing the results, the camera poses were computed using our trained networks from a simulated video consisting of 450 frames which were never observed by the networks during training or validation. The outcome for the distance traveled by the colonoscope camera along the Z direction is shown in Fig. 4, which demonstrates the high performance of the modified GoogLeNet trained by gray scale images.

4.2 Validation Using a Colonoscopy Phantom

Prior to validating our trained network on actual colonoscopy frames which were obtained from patients, we estimated the camera pose when colonoscope traveled back and forth in a straight phantom. It started from a start point, which represented as frame (s) in Fig. 5, and returned to the same place frame (e). Results for the distance traveled by camera in Z direction from different networks are shown in Fig. 5. The modified GoogLeNet which was trained by frames shows the lowest drift in comparison to SfM (D2) and the AlexNet when it was trained by optical flow (D1).

4.3 Application to Actual Colonoscopy Video

Actual colonoscopy videos from different parts of colons were chosen, specifically when the camera moved back and forth (a common practice during colonoscopy) to

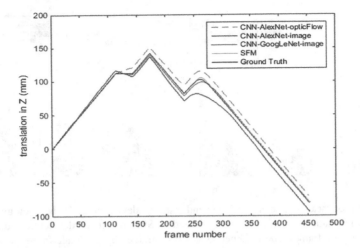

Fig. 4. The comparison for generalization of camera motion estimation by AlexNet when optical flow and frames were used for training and GoogLeNet when frames were used for training on a dataset that has not been seen before. Here, GoogLeNet shows better performance.

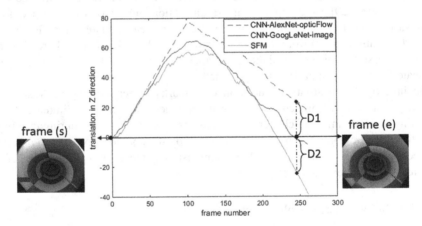

Fig. 5. Distance traveled by camera in the Z direction estimated by modified AlexNet, GoogLeNet and SfM (D1 and D2 represent the drift in camera motion estimation by modified AlexNet and SfM respectively), the GoogLeNet trained by frames shows very low drift.

allow validation. We estimated the distance camera traveled in the Z direction by SfM, and our CNN methods. Figure 6 represents a qualitative evaluation of the methods in the Z coordinate. During one typical examination, the colonoscope was moved back and forth during withdrawal (video in supplementary materials). The graph shows the estimation of Z coordinate along the center line for three different methods (see legend). The image inserts compares different frames that are estimated to be from the same Z location. The orange frame 54 (left insert) was visually closer to frame 166 (top magenta on right inserts) than to frame 141 (green image on right insert), suggesting

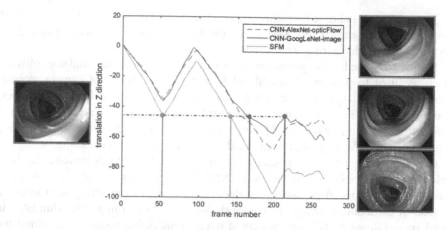

Fig. 6. The camera translation in the Z direction estimated by modified AlexNet, GoogLeNet and SfM on an actual colonoscopy video frames. Frames in orange, green and magenta are chosen to be from same Z height, but we visually understand that the closest frame to orange is the first magenta on the right inset. The modified GoogLeNet trained by grayscale frames and modified AlexNet trained by optical flow are showing better results in comparison to SfM. (color figure online)

that the CNN-based method is more accurate than the previous SfM approach. In addition, the CNN method estimated that frame 215 (magenta, bottom right insert) was also at the same location as frame 54 (orange left insert), which visually matches, whereas a drift was observed for the SfM method.

5 Discussion and Conclusion

In this paper, we presented a method to estimate the relative camera pose with six DoF from actual colonoscopy video frames. We used two separate new approaches: one modified and trained GoogLeNet using two consecutive grayscale frames as input; the other modified and trained AlexNet and used the optical flow pattern (SIFT flow) and consecutive frames (for the sake of comparison) as input. The networks, trained by simulated data were validated on simulated and actual colonoscopy frames. Our results, which are presented in Fig. 3 showed that the network which was trained with two consecutive frames could outperform the one which was trained by optical flow. In addition, modified GoogLeNet which was trained by frames had better performance in generalizing results for frames that had not been observed in training or validation stage in comparison to the one which was trained by optical flow, as it shown in Fig. 4. Some colonoscopy frames are feature-poor, thus it is hard to find accurate matches between frames, and that rendering the conventional SfM approach is inaccurate. In contrast, CNN-based approach is more robust to these issues, and resulting in higher accuracy Fig. 3.

The computational time for estimating relative camera pose from a trained network was 0.1 s on average, whereas SfM with a bundle adjustment as optimizer took three seconds when Matlab scripts were used.

In this study, we had the ground truth for camera pose from the simulator software, which we used to generate thousands of frames with a variety of camera motions incorporating translation and rotation for training and validation. Previously, others used a robot hand, magnetic sensor [14] or SfM algorithm to estimate camera pose as ground truth to train a network [15]. Any error in calibrating the sensor or estimating camera pose by SfM as ground truth could result in false data for training.

Our results on actual colonoscopy which presented in Fig. 6 indicate the high performance of CNNs in comparison to SfM for estimating the distance in the Z direction that a colonoscope camera traveled in returning to a previously seen location.

One of the main challenges in our work was transfer learning from simulated to actual frames domain. Although we could obtain remarkable results using simulated data and pre-trained networks, as a part of our future work we aim at implementing domain transfer method to improve our current results. We also investigate the performance of other networks such as visual geometry group (VGG) and will propose our network to estimate colonoscope pose.

References

1. Australian Institute of Health and Welfare. http://www.aihw.gov.au/
2. World Health Organization (WHO). Fact sheet # 297: Cancer. http://www.who.int/mediacentre/factsheets/fs297/en/
3. Hewett, D.G., Kahi, C.J., Rex, D.K.: Does colonoscopy work? J. Natl. Compr. Cancer Netw. JNCCN **8**, 67–76 (2010). quiz 77
4. Cotton, P.B., Williams, C.B.: Practical Gastrointestinal Endoscopy. Wiley-Blackwell, Oxford (2008)
5. Puerto-Souza, G.A., Staranowicz, A.N., Bell, C.S., Valdastri, P., Mariottini, G.-L.: A comparative study of ego-motion estimation algorithms for teleoperated robotic endoscopes. In: Luo, X., Reichl, T., Mirota, D., Soper, T. (eds.) CARE 2014. LNCS, vol. 8899, pp. 64–76. Springer, Cham (2014). doi:10.1007/978-3-319-13410-9_7
6. Liu, J., Subramanian, K.R., Yoo, T.S.: A robust method to track colonoscopy videos with non-informative images. Int. J. Comput. Assist. Radiol. Surg. **8**, 575–592 (2013)
7. Armin, M.A., Chetty, G., De Visser, H., Dumas, C., Grimpen, F., Salvado, O.: Automated visibility map of the internal colon surface from colonoscopy video. Int. J. Comput. Assist. Radiol. Surg. **11**, 1599–1610 (2016)
8. Rai, L., Helferty, J.P., Higgins, W.E.: Combined video tracking and image-video registration for continuous bronchoscopic guidance. Int. J. Comput. Assist. Radiol. Surg. **3**, 315–329 (2008)
9. Bao, G., Pahlavan, K., Mi, L.: Hybrid localization of microrobotic endoscopic capsule inside small intestine by data fusion of vision and RF sensors. IEEE Sens. J. **15**, 2669–2678 (2015)
10. Krizhevsky, A., Sutskever, I., Hinton, G.E.: Imagenet classification with deep convolutional neural networks. In: Advances in Neural Information Processing Systems, pp. 1097–1105 (2012)
11. Aubry, M., Maturana, D., Efros, A.A., Russell, B.C., Sivic, J.: Seeing 3D Chairs: Exemplar Part-Based 2D-3D Alignment Using a Large Dataset of CAD Models, June 2014

12. Dosovitskiy, A., Fischery, P., Ilg, E., Hazirbas, C., Golkov, V., van der Smagt, P., Cremers, D., Brox, T.: Flownet: learning optical flow with convolutional networks. In: 2015 IEEE International Conference on Computer Vision (ICCV), pp. 2758–2766. IEEE (2015)
13. Zhou, T., Krähenbühl, P., Aubry, M., Huang, Q., Efros, A.A.: Learning Dense Correspondence via 3D-guided Cycle Consistency. ArXiv Prepr. arXiv:1604.05383 (2016)
14. Bell, C.S., Obstein, K.L., Valdastri, P.: Image partitioning and illumination in image-based pose detection for teleoperated flexible endoscopes. Artif. Intell. Med. **59**, 185–196 (2013)
15. Kendall, A., Grimes, M., Cipolla, R.: Convolutional networks for real-time 6-DOF camera relocalization. Proceedings of the International Conference on Computer Vision (ICCV) (2015)
16. Su, H., Qi, C.R., Li, Y., Guibas, L.J.: Render for CNN: viewpoint estimation in images using CNNs trained with rendered 3D model views. In: Proceedings of the IEEE International Conference on Computer Vision, pp. 2686–2694 (2015)
17. Mayer, N., Ilg, E., Hausser, P., Fischer, P., Cremers, D., Dosovitskiy, A., Brox, T.: A large dataset to train convolutional networks for disparity, optical flow, and scene flow estimation. In: Presented at the Proceedings of the IEEE Conference on Computer Vision and Pattern Recognition (2016)
18. Armin, M.A., De Visser, H., Chetty, G., Dumas, C., Conlan, D., Grimpen, F., Salvado, O.: Visibility map: a new method in evaluation quality of optical colonoscopy. In: Navab, N., Hornegger, J., Wells, W.M., Frangi, A.F. (eds.) MICCAI 2015. LNCS, vol. 9349, pp. 396–404. Springer, Cham (2015). doi:10.1007/978-3-319-24553-9_49
19. Liu, C., Yuen, J., Torralba, A., Sivic, J., Freeman, W.T.: SIFT flow: dense correspondence across different scenes. In: Forsyth, D., Torr, P., Zisserman, A. (eds.) ECCV 2008. LNCS, vol. 5304, pp. 28–42. Springer, Heidelberg (2008). doi:10.1007/978-3-540-88690-7_3
20. Armin, M.A., Chetty, G., Jurgen, F., De Visser, H., Dumas, C., Fazlollahi, A., Grimpen, F., Salvado, O.: Uninformative frame detection in colonoscopy through motion, edge and color features. In: Luo, X., Reichl, T., Reiter, A., Mariottini, G.-L. (eds.) CARE 2015. LNCS, vol. 9515, pp. 153–162. Springer, Cham (2016). doi:10.1007/978-3-319-29965-5_15
21. Huynh, D.Q.: Metrics for 3D rotations: comparison and analysis. J. Math. Imaging Vis. **35**, 155–164 (2009)
22. Vedaldi, A., Lenc, K.: MatConvNet: Convolutional Neural Networks for MATLAB (2015)
23. De Visser, H., Passenger, J., Conlan, D., Russ, C., Hellier, D., Cheng, M., Acosta, O., Ourselin, S., Salvado, O.: Developing a next generation colonoscopy simulator. Int. J. Image Graph. **10**, 203–217 (2010)

Motion Vector for Outlier Elimination in Feature Matching and Its Application in SLAM Based Laparoscopic Tracking

Cheng Wang[1]([⊠]), Masahiro Oda[2], Yuichiro Hayashi[2], Kazunari Misawa[3], Holger Roth[2], and Kensaku Mori[2]

[1] Graduate School of Information Science, Nagoya University, Nagoya, Japan
{chwang,moda,yhayashi,rothhr}@mori.m.is.nagoya-u.ac.jp
[2] Graduate School of Informatics, Nagoya University, Nagoya, Japan
kensaku@is.nagoya-u.ac.jp
[3] Aichi Cancer Center Hospital, Nagoya, Japan
misawakzn@aichi-cc.jp

Abstract. This paper presents a motion vector-based method to detect and remove the outlier of the matched feature point in laparoscopic images. Feature point detected on organ surface in laparoscopic images plays an important role not only in laparoscopic tracking but also in organ surface shape reconstruction. However, many factors such as the deformation of the organ or the movement of the surgical tools result to the outliers in matched feature points, thus the feature point based tracking and reconstruction will have larger errors. Traditional methods use these points either directly (inside a RANSAC scheme) or after a prior knowledge of compensation, which may lead to larger error in tracking and reconstruction. We introduce the motion vector (MV) based method to detect outliers among the matched feature points. MV is originally used in the compression of the video streams, we exploit it to detect the movement of one feature point in different video frames. The outliers of feature point can be detected by enforcing a direction constraint with its MV. Our method had been implement under a SLAM-based framework for laparoscopic tracking, we modified the map management of SLAM for better laparoscopic tracking. The experimental results showed that our method effectively detects and removes the outliers without any prior knowledge; the average precision rate in image pairs was 95.9%.

Keywords: Laparoscopic tracking · Motion vector · SLAM

1 Introduction

In recent years, minimally invasive surgery (MIS) has became more popular due to its benefit to patients. However, MIS has drawbacks such as the limited view to surgeons. Therefore, endoscopic surgery navigation systems are used to make MIS processes safe and effective [1]. However, traditional endoscopic navigation needs additional equipment such as optical or magnetic trackers, that make

© Springer International Publishing AG 2017
M.J. Cardoso et al. (Eds.): CARE/CLIP 2017, LNCS 10550, pp. 60–69, 2017.
DOI: 10.1007/978-3-319-67543-5_6

the endoscopic surgery navigation systems complex. To make the endoscope navigation system simple, the endoscope pose obtaining from the endoscopic videos instead of using additional equipment has been explored [2].

Visual simultaneous localization and mapping $(VSLAM)$ is an approach for camera localization and 3D reconstruction. It has been introduced into laparoscopic navigation since 2006 [1,3,4]. However, even though breakthroughs have been made in recent years, many questions remain unsolved. For example, organ deformation may increase the error of laparoscopic tracking and in-vivo reconstruction.

Previous research [2] assumed rigid (or generally rigid) environments that all matched feature points are used for the estimation of laparoscope posture and 3D environments. This may result in the large difference comparing with real posture of laparoscope. Yang et al. established an online estimation of tissue deformation by exploiting a periodic motion model to estimate the organ's deformation [5]. They kept the estimation of the feature points detected on the organ surface using a filter-based SLAM. However, at least two assumptions were made: periodic organ motion, and as few other deformations as possible. A short observation for organ deformation with static camera is also needed before tracking. Clooins et al. exploited the prior information of organ shape for 3D tracking reconstruction without feature detecting in their work, and showed a good performance [6]. Mahmoud et al. extended the density of SLAM's map by enforcing cross-correlation on newly selected frames [7]. Their results showed that the reconstructed maps have higher density than the original SLAM with a higher RMSE value comparing with the segmented preoperative CT scans. Gustavo et al. exploited a HMA-based method to improve the performance of feature matching in MIS scenarios [8]. However, their work may be helpful in the reconstruction of the organ shape while it may behaves poor in real time tracking of the laparoscope.

Since previous methods use matched feature points for laparoscopic tracking, the laparoscopic tracking might fail due to the outliers existed in matched feature points. To remove these feature points, we use a motion vector-based method to judge the motion of the matched feature points. Motion vector (MV) was previously proposed [9] to detect object's movement within a SLAM solution. A voting procedure to determine the camera direction and a filtering procedure to reduce feature points were used. However, due to the difference between indoor/outdoor scenes and laparoscope scenes, the procedure we used is more strict.

Our main contribution is find a new method for the detection of the outlier existed in the matched feature points during laparoscopic tracking by the combination of the pure translational motion and the MV of the matched features. Different from the traditional method, our MV-based method detect the outliers by enforcing the direction constraint on the displacement of the feature point after the detection of eipolar constraint. The outliers in matched feature points can be detected and removed without any prior knowledge, this is quite different from the traditional method [5,9]. We explain this procedure in Sect. 2.

The performance of our method were shown in Sect. 3, the difference in tracked images and trajectories could be found.

2   Methodology

The goal of our method is to detect the outlier in matched feature points. To achieve this goal, we use three steps: (1) initial motion estimation of two images; (2) feature point selection using motion vector (MV); (3) motion refine using optimization. These three steps check the matched feature point not only with the traditional epipolar constraint, but also with the characteristic of pure transformation. Therefore, the small displacement of feature point caused by different factors can be detected and removed. We introduce the proposed feature point selection method into the ORB-SLAM to improve the tracking quality during laparoscopic tracking. The flowchart of the system implement with our method is shown in Fig. 1.

2.1   MV-Based Method for Motion Estimation

Initial Motion Estimation. Our method starts from the estimation of the motion between two images. Assume that two images at the time (m) and (n) are obtained, they are denoted as $I^{(m)}$ and $I^{(n)}$. The two images should have overlapping views so that enough feature points can be matched and used for motion estimation. Then the ORB feature is used to extract and match feature point in $I^{(m)}$ and $I^{(n)}$ [10]. After the feature matching procedure, a set of corresponding feature points $C^{(m,n)} = \left\{ x_i^{(m)} \leftrightarrow x_i^{(n)} \mid x_i^{(m)} \in P^{(m)}, x_i^{(n)} \in P^{(n)} \right\}$ are obtained, where $P^{(m)}$ are the extracted feature points in $I^{(m)}$ and $P^{(n)}$ are the extracted feature points in $I^{(n)}$, respectively.

With the use of the matched feature points $C^{(m,n)}$, an initial fundamental matrix $F^{(m,n)}$ can be computed using the eight-point algorithm with utilization

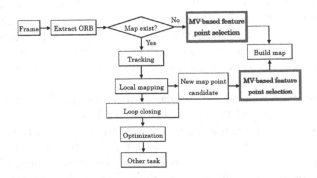

Fig. 1. ORB-SLAM flowchart implementing MV-based feature point selection procedure: tracking is used to track new frame; local mapping is used to create more map point; optimization is used for posture optimization. (Color figure online)

of a RANSAC algorithm [11] for outlier exclusion. The initial fundamental matrix $F^{(m,n)}$ gives an inlier corresponding set in the matched feature points:

$$C^{(m,n)'} = \left\{ x_i^{(m)} \leftrightarrow x_i^{(n)} \mid x_i^{(m)} \leftrightarrow x_i^{(n)} \subset C^{(m,n)}, (x_i^{(m)})^{\mathrm{T}} F^{(m,n)} x_i^{(n)} < \epsilon \right\} \quad (1)$$

where ϵ is an error threshold. The fundamental matrix $F^{(m,n)}$ is also used to calculate the essential matrix $E^{(m,n)}$ using $E^{(m,n)} = K^{\mathrm{T}} F^{(m,n)} K$, where K is the intrinsic parameter. The essential matrix $E^{(m,n)}$ is decomposed to obtain the transformation between two images [11].

After this step, a subset of the corresponding feature points $C^{(m,n)'}$ and the transformation $T^{(m,n)} = \begin{bmatrix} sR^{(m,n)} & t^{(m,n)} \\ 0 & 1 \end{bmatrix}$ are obtained, where $R^{(m,n)}$, $t^{(m,n)}$ are the rotation and translation between two images, respectively. For adjacent frames in laparoscope video, the scaling s is set to 1.

MV-Based Method for Feature Point Selection. Unlike the other outdoor/indoor scenes, the in-vivo scenes are more complex and challenging due to the influence of factors such as the deformation of the organ, the movement of the forceps and so on. To improve the camera localization accuracy, only the inlier feature points are used.

To distinguish the matched feature points, we first rotate the feature points in $\mathbf{x}_i^{(m)}$ to a new position by using

$$\mathbf{x}_i^{(m)'} = sKR^{(m,n)}K^{-1}\mathbf{x}_i^{(m)} \quad (2)$$

where $\mathbf{x}_i^{(m)'}$ is the new position of $\mathbf{x}_i^{(m)}$ after rotation $R^{(m,n)}$ and scaling s. With this equation, the motion of the feature point can be changed to pure translation. Motion vectors (MVs) of feature points can be expressed as $\mathbf{x}_i^{(n)} - e$ and $\mathbf{x}_i^{(n)} - \mathbf{x}_i^{(m)'}$, where e is the epipole on image $I^{(n)}$. For the pure translational motion, vectors $\mathbf{x}_i^{(n)} - e$ and $\mathbf{x}_i^{(n)} - \mathbf{x}_i^{(m)'}$ are collinear [11]. However, in the abdominal cavity, due to the influence of factors mentioned above, these two vectors become non-collinear and the angle α is not $0°$ or $180°$. Examples are shown in Figs. 2 and 3.

However, since the displacement caused by the additional motion is small, these feature point can't be detected by using constraint such as epipolar constraint or symmetric transfer error. To detect these outliers out, the angle of the motion vectors is used. The feature point is identified as outlier if

$$|cos(\alpha)| = \left| \frac{\left(\mathbf{x}_i^{(n)} - e \right)}{\left| \mathbf{x}_i^{(n)} - e \right|} \cdot \frac{\left(\mathbf{x}_i^{(n)} - \mathbf{x}_i^{(m)'} \right)}{\left| \mathbf{x}_i^{(n)} - \mathbf{x}_i^{(m)'} \right|} \right| < \lambda, \quad (3)$$

where λ is an threshold; otherwise, the feature point is identified as inlier. The inlier feature points are selected as the input for the motion refine procedure.

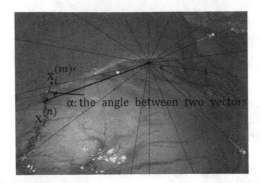

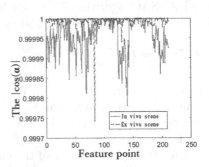

Fig. 2. An example of MV in laparoscope image. The red arrows show corresponding points $\mathbf{x}^{(m)'}$ and $\mathbf{x}_i^{(n)}$, while the black lines show $\mathbf{x}_i^{(n)}$ and the epipole e. Feature points of inliers should show the correspondence as the green arrows while the outlier is the red arrows [11]. (Color figure online)

Fig. 3. The matched feature points and the cosine value of the angle α. We calculate the $|cos(\alpha)|$ in two scene: one is the ex vivo scene (blue line) and the other one is the in vivo abdominal scene exists both the non-rigid motion and rigid motion (red line). The average of $|cos(\alpha)|$ is closer to 1 in ex vivo scene while the abdominal scene is not. (Color figure online)

We can obtain a subset of $\boldsymbol{C}^{(m,n)'}$ marked

$$\boldsymbol{C}^{(m,n)''} = \left\{ \boldsymbol{x}_i^{(m)} \leftrightarrow \boldsymbol{x}_i^{(n)} \middle| \left| \frac{\left(\boldsymbol{x}_i^{(n)} - e\right)}{\left|\boldsymbol{x}_i^{(n)} - e\right|} \cdot \frac{\left(\boldsymbol{x}_i^{(n)} - \boldsymbol{x}_i^{'(m)}\right)}{\left|\boldsymbol{x}_i^{(n)} - \boldsymbol{x}_i^{'(m)}\right|} \right| \geq \lambda \right\}. \tag{4}$$

Motion Refine. The motion refine procedure is used to optimize the transformation of two images using the inlier feature points. The transformation is optimized by minimizing the reprojection error using

$$\mathrm{T}_r^{*(m,n)} = \arg\min_{\mathrm{T}_r^{(m,n)}} \sum_j \rho \left\| \boldsymbol{x}_j^{(n)} - proj\left(\mathrm{T}_r^{(m,n)}, \boldsymbol{X}_j^{(n)}\right) \right\|, \tag{5}$$

where $\mathbf{X}_j^{(n)}$ is the j-th recovered world coordinate of the feature point $\mathbf{x}_j^{(n)}$, *proj* is the projection function projecting $\mathbf{X}_j^{(n)}$ onto $I^{(m)}$ [9,12], ρ is the Huber influence function [13].

Finally, we can obtain an optimized transformation $\mathrm{T}_r^{*(m,n)}$ between two images and a subset of matched feature points satisfying Eq. 4.

2.2   Application in ORB-SLAM Based Tracking

ORB-SLAM is an ORB feature-based SLAM framework and superior to other visual SLAM methods such as PTAM [12] and EKF-SLAM [3,13]. The feasibility of ORB-SLAM in endoscope surgery navigation has been proved [7].

We implemented our method on the ORB-SLAM. The flowchart of the modified ORB-SLAM is shown in Fig. 1, where the red part is the implementation of our method. We explain in details in the following parts.

Detection in Map Initialization. We modify the map initialization procedure of ORB-SLAM to initialize the map using fundamental matrix. The matched feature points should pass the test of motion model as well as our MV-based detection before they are used in map point creation.

Detection of New Map Points. New map points are created in the local mapping procedure of the ORB-SLAM. Feature points in the selected frames (called key frames) are matched and used to create new map points. New map points are created after the matched feature points pass the test of epipolar constraint and our MV-based approach.

Key Frame Management. Our MV-based method can detect the outlier of feature points especially observing the non-rigid motion. This can decrease the number of map points, and finally may resulting in the failure of laparoscopic tracking. To avoid this, we lower the threshold in the key frame selection to allow more key frames are used in building of the map. In actual implementation, we create the key frame every two frames and cull them if we have tracked enough points.

3 Experiments and Results

We validated our approach with in-vivo laparoscope videos. The videos recorded a task of exploring the abdominal cavity with a resolution of 640×480 pixels at 25 fps. The deformation in laparoscope videos were not too large [14]. We set the number of the ORB feature points in each frame to 2000, and the threshold λ was set to the mean value of $|cos(\alpha)|$ in rigid scene.

3.1 Detection Rate in Image Pairs

We saved the frames used in the map initialization during laparoscopic tracking. The ground truth is created by annotating the matched feature points manually. The matched feature points were marked true if it is found as outlier, and were marked false if it is found as inlier. The type of matched feature point is judged according to their neighbor and position. Table 1 shows the false positive (FP) rate, precision rate and recall rate of feature points of our method.

Table 1. Detection rate of proposed method in laparoscope images

Index	TP	FP	FP rate [%]	Precision rate [%]	Recall rate [%]	Miss rate [%]
1	252	17	47.1	93.7	100	0
2	129	4	13.7	96.9	100	0
3	99	6	31.6	94.3	100	0
4	88	17	5.5	98.9	100	0

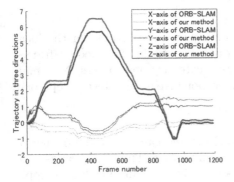

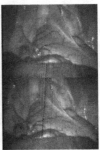

Fig. 4. Comparison of trajectory between our method and the original SLAM method. We can see the differences in two trajectories as frame changes.

Fig. 5. Matched feature points in the key frames. Green and yellow lines show matched feature points of inlier and outlier, respectively. We have removed the yellow lines to show clearly in the right figure. (Color figure online)

3.2 Performance in Laparoscopic Video

We used the laparoscope videos mentioned above as the input of our system. The videos can be processed in real time. We obtained 5087 map points with the original ORB-SLAM and 3807 map points using SLAM implemented with our method. A comparison of trajectories between our method and the original SLAM was shown in Fig. 4. Due to no ground truth of laparoscope trajectory in real clinical scene, we only showed the difference of two methods in three directions in this figure: x-axis is the right direction, y-axis is the down direction, and z-axis is the front direction, respectively. We used the median depth of the first frame to make the trajectory under the same scale with that of the ORB-SLAM [13]. The matched feature points are shown in Figs. 5 and 6. Matched feature points are connected by yellow lines if they are judged as outliers while feature points are connected by green line if they are judged as inliers. The performance of our method in the local mapping procedure of SLAM is also validated. Figure 6 shows the matched feature points between the key frames. Some mismatched feature points together with feature points observing the non-rigid motion were detected by our method while they are poorly detected by the original ORB-SLAM.

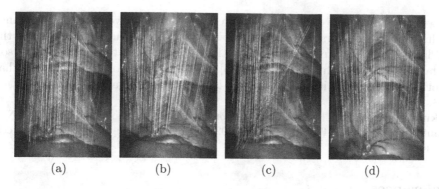

(a)   (b)   (c)   (d)

Fig. 6. Matched feature points in key frames. Green and yellow lines show feature point in rigid and non-rigid motion area, respectively. (a)–(c) pairs show good results, (c) shows the mismatched feature point. (d) shows poor result caused by wrong motion estimation. (Color figure online)

4   Discussion

We confirm that the proposed method performs good in detecting and removing the outlier feature points during vision-based laparoscopic tracking. Our method exploit the characteristic of pure translation to find the outlier of the match, feature points with small displacement can be found using our method while they can't be detected by traditional method.

Figure 6(c) demonstrates that the mismatched feature points can be detected. This is because the MVs of the mismatched feature points also showing large angles. The mismatched feature points can also decrease the accuracy of the tracking.

Table 1 shows a comparison of our method and the map initialization procedure of ORB-SLAM. Our method can detect the outlier feature points even though after the test of ORB-SLAM initialization procedure. From this table, we can see our method outperform the map initialization procedure of ORB-SLAM.

However, since our method based on the estimated transformation between two images, the accuracy of our method depends on the estimated transformation. If the transformation is wrongly estimated, our method can't eliminate the outlier correctly. An undesirable result was shown in the fourth pair of Fig. 6. This result is caused by the incorrect transformation between two images.

In our experiment, the threshold λ is set according to the rigid scene. However, the value of λ can have an influence on the robust of the tracking. Too large or too small will cause the failure of the tracking, so the relationship between the λ and the tracking quality should be studied in the future.

5   Conclusion and Future Work

We proposed a motion vector-based method to detect the outlier feature points in laparoscopic video. The proposed method uses the transformation estimated between two images to distinguish feature points and achieved good performance both in the image pairs and in SLAM-based tracking. Future work contains the validation of the laparoscope posture estimated by our method, the comparison with other system such as RS-SLAM [15], and the discussion with surgeons that whether the accuracy is satisfactory for laparoscope navigation.

Acknowledgments. This work was supported by the MEXT, the JSPS KAKENHI Grant Numbers 25242047, 26108006, 26560255, 17H00869. We thanks to our lab colleagues for their help.

References

1. Baumhauer, M., Feuerstein, M., Meinzer, H.P., Rassweiler, J.: Navigation in endoscopic soft tissue surgery: perspectives and limitations. J. Endourol. **22**(4), 751–766 (2008)
2. Grasa, O.G., Bernal, E., Casado, S., Gil, I., Montiel, J.M.M.: Visual SLAM for handheld monocular endoscope. IEEE Trans. Med. Imaging **33**(1), 135–146 (2014)
3. Civera, J., Grasa, O.G., Davison, A.J., Montiel, J.M.M.: 1-Point RANSAC for extended kalman filtering: application to real-time structure from motion and visual odometry. J. Field Robot. **27**(5), 609–631 (2010)
4. Mountney, P., Stoyanov, D., Davison, A., Yang, G.-Z.: Simultaneous stereoscope localization and soft-tissue mapping for minimal invasive surgery. In: Larsen, R., Nielsen, M., Sporring, J. (eds.) MICCAI 2006. LNCS, vol. 4190, pp. 347–354. Springer, Heidelberg (2006). doi:10.1007/11866565_43
5. Mountney, P., Yang, G.-Z.: Motion compensated SLAM for image guided surgery. In: Jiang, T., Navab, N., Pluim, J.P.W., Viergever, M.A. (eds.) MICCAI 2010. LNCS, vol. 6362, pp. 496–504. Springer, Heidelberg (2010). doi:10.1007/978-3-642-15745-5_61
6. Collins, T., Bartoli, A., Bourdel, N., Canis, M.: Robust, real-time, dense and deformable 3D organ tracking in laparoscopic videos. In: Ourselin, S., Joskowicz, L., Sabuncu, M.R., Unal, G., Wells, W. (eds.) MICCAI 2016. LNCS, vol. 9900, pp. 404–412. Springer, Cham (2016). doi:10.1007/978-3-319-46720-7_47
7. Mahmoud, N., Cirauqui, I., Hostettler, A., Doignon, C., Soler, L., Marescaux, J., Montiel, J.M.M.: ORBSLAM-based endoscope tracking and 3D reconstruction. arXiv preprint (2016). arXiv:1608.08149
8. Puerto-Souza, G.A., Mariottini, G.-L.: A fast and accurate feature-matching algorithm for minimally-invasive endoscopic images. IEEE Trans. Med. Imaging **32**(7), 1201–1214 (2013)
9. Li, W., Song, D.: Featureless motion vector-based simultaneous localization, planar surface extraction, and moving obstacle tracking. In: Akin, H.L., Amato, N.M., Isler, V., van der Stappen, A.F. (eds.) Algorithmic Foundations of Robotics XI. STAR, vol. 107, pp. 245–261. Springer, Cham (2015). doi:10.1007/978-3-319-16595-0_15
10. Rublee, E., Rabaud, V., Konolige, K., Bradski, G.: ORB: an efficient alternative to SIFT or SURF. In: 2011 IEEE International Conference on Computer Vision (ICCV), pp. 2564–2571 (2011)
11. Hartley, R., Zisserman, A.: Multiple View Geometry in Computer Vision. Cambridge University Press, Cambridge (2003)

12. Klein, G., Murray, D.: Parallel tracking and mapping for small AR workspaces. In: 6th IEEE and ACM International Symposium on Mixed and Augmented Reality, ISMAR 2007, pp. 225–234 (2007)
13. Mur-Artal, R., Montiel, J.M.M., Tardos, J.D.: ORB-SLAM: a versatile and accurate monocular SLAM system. IEEE Trans. Robot. **31**(5), 1147–1163 (2015)
14. Mountney, P., Stoyanov, D., Yang, G.Z.: Three-dimensional tissue deformation recovery and tracking. IEEE Signal Process. Magaz. **27**(4), 14–24 (2010)
15. Lee, G.H., Fraundorfer, F., Pollefeys, M.: RS-SLAM: RANSAC sampling for visual FastSLAM. In: International Conference on Intelligent Robots and Systems, pp. 1655–1660 (2011)

Image-Based Smoke Detection
in Laparoscopic Videos

Andreas Leibetseder[✉], Manfred Jürgen Primus, Stefan Petscharnig,
and Klaus Schoeffmann

Institute of Information Technology, Alpen-Adria University,
9020 Klagenfurt, Austria
{aleibets,mprimus,spetsch,ks}@itec.aau.at

Abstract. The development and improper removal of smoke during
minimally invasive surgery (MIS) can considerably impede a patient's
treatment, while additionally entailing serious deleterious health effects.
Hence, state-of-the-art surgical procedures employ smoke evacuation systems, which often still are activated manually by the medical staff or less
commonly operate automatically utilizing industrial, highly-specialized
and operating room (OR) approved sensors. As an alternate approach,
video analysis can be used to take on said detection process – a topic
not yet much researched in aforementioned context. In order to advance
in this sector, we propose utilizing an image-based smoke classification
task on a pre-trained convolutional neural network (CNN). We provide
a custom data set of over 30 000 laparoscopic smoke/non-smoke images,
part of which served as training data for GoogLeNet-based [41] CNN
models. To be able to compare our research for evaluation, we separately
developed a non-CNN classifier based on observing the saturation channel of a sample picture in the HSV color space. While the deep learning
approaches yield excellent results with Receiver Operating Characteristic (ROC) curves enclosing areas of over 0.98, the computationally much
less costly analysis of an image's saturation histogram under certain circumstances can, surprisingly, as well be a good indicator for smoke with
areas under the curves (AUCs) of around 0.92–0.97.

Keywords: Smoke detection · Endoscopy · Image processing · Deep
learning

1 Introduction

Substantial advances in health care technology over the recent decades enabled
minimally invasive surgery (MIS), i.e. medical operations inflicting as little as
possible physical trauma upon patients, to become common practice in the clinical community. Nowadays, some surgical interventions almost exclusively are
performed via MIS [46], such as the cholecystectomy procedure for attending
gallbladder conditions. Regarding the technology applied in such or similar situations, physicians rely on video-monitoring their treatment of a patient's internal

© Springer International Publishing AG 2017
M.J. Cardoso et al. (Eds.): CARE/CLIP 2017, LNCS 10550, pp. 70–87, 2017.
DOI: 10.1007/978-3-319-67543-5_7

anatomy – a modus operandi achievable by introducing a high definition camera or *endoscope* in addition to a variety of instruments through bodily orifices. The corresponding medical field, namely endoscopy, is sub-categorized by considering the insertion locality of said video device, which may be natural apertures such as nose (rhinoscopy), ear (otoscopy), anus (anoscopy) etc. or deliberately created incisions used in order to examine interior cavities of joints (arthroscopy), thorax (thoracoscopy) as well as of the most frequently inspected abdomen – a zone treatable via a broad number of procedures that comprise the field of *laparoscopy*, constituting the main focus of this study.

Many laparoscopic actions require severing tissue, which can create open wounds causing internal bleeding, a matter which usually needs to be tended to urgently. This typically is accomplished by suturing, i.e. sewing parts of the affected tissue back together and thereby helping natural hemostasis, as well as cauterization, that is using electrically heated or laser instruments[1] in order to mitigate or stop the hemorrhage. The latter either can be applied during dissection as to prevent aforementioned effects or afterwards in an attempt to seal afflicted regions. In any case, it is estimated that tissue cauterization is applied in well over 90% of all surgical procedures, generating yet another undesirable side-effect: a gaseous mixture consisting of 95% water and 5% chemical, biological as well as physical by-products [32] – materials comprising a *surgical smoke plume*. Potentially harmful contained substances like toxins, viruses or bacteria as well as ultrafine particulate matter renders exposure to such an entity a possibly serious health risk for both medical staff and patients, as is indicated in a great amount of scientific documents [5,10,14,21,34,37,43]. Thus, the necessity of removing surgical smoke swiftly and safely after its creation seems imperative in modern medicine, yet involved hazards still are underestimated, which can cause bad decisions like releasing corresponding fumes into the operating room (OR) air[2], a not uncommon practice according to Sahaf et al. [5].

Proper smoke evacuation on the other hand is accomplished via OR-approved suction systems that typically are activated manually by the medical staff, in case cauterization is conducted. However, this particular action can easily be forgotten or neglected, potentially leading up to a point, in which the operating staff's view onto the currently treated body parts is severely obstructed by smoke – Fig. 1 demonstrates such situations by portraying three laparoscopic scenes that depict the emergence of smoke in various intensities.

In addition to the inconvenience of requiring manual control, smoke evacuators designed for laparoscopic utilization must be able to keep the abdominal cavity from collapsing during the suction process, which is achieved by using a medical grade insufflation gas[3] [7], entailing additional budget expenses to clinical institutions. Thus, handling a smoke evacuator inefficiently, which very likely happens many times during critical situations like surgeries, comes at a price. Naturally, automatic evacuation would represent an optimal solution for

---

[1] Temperatures range from about 100°–1200° Celsius.

[2] This effect is achieved by opening the stopcock of the laparoscopic port.

[3] In laparoscopy usually carbon dioxide (CO_2) is used [35].

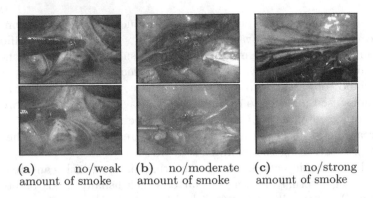

(a)   no/weak   (b) no/moderate   (c)   no/strong
amount of smoke   amount of smoke   amount of smoke

Fig. 1. Comparison of non-smoke vs. smoke images with different effect intensities.

both the nuisance of manual evacuator operation and the possibility of wasting valuable resources. Systems targeting similar goals have already been proposed, albeit all of them pursuing the rather naive methodology of commencing smoke removal whenever a cauterization instrument is activated [12,13,42]. Considering such a procedure fairly excessive and hardware restrictive, we argue that it is possible to construct more fine-grained, universal systems by detecting smoke via *image analysis* accurately and in real-time. Therefore, we formulate the research question behind our work as follows:

Q Can image-based analysis of endoscopic videos be leveraged as to reliably recognize the emergence of smoke in real-time?

Our proposed strategies to answer **Q** in general fall into the category of *binary classification tasks* – we develop a simple image saturation based histogram thresholding algorithm and compare its performance to two state-of-the-art CNN-based approaches.

The remainder of this work is subdivided into four sections: related work described in following Sect. 2, a detailed account of the methodology we apply in Sect. 3, evaluation results containing performance as well as runtime analyses in Sect. 4 and a concluding Sect. 5 highlighting our scientific contributions.

2   Related Work

Today classification utilizing CNNs is already commonly used in the medical field – research on the topic can be found dating back to the mid-1990s, where for example Sahiner et al. developed a three-layer CNN approach to be able to differentiate between normal tissue and abnormal areas (mass) when analyzing mammograms achieving a ROC AUC of 0.87 [40]. Further work using CNNs on computerized tomographic (CT) and Magnetic Resonance Imaging (MRI) images include Li et al. [30], who are detecting five different lung states related to interstitial lung diseases with 0.8 precision, 0.9 recall for each of them.

Conducting research in the same area, Anthimopoulos et al. [6] defined seven classes and they were able to outperform the former as well as other state-of-the-art methods. Moreover, Yan et al. [48] developed a multi-stage deep learning framework utilizing a CNN structure to automatically determine characteristics of different body parts, altogether exceeding recall, precision and F1 score of standard CNNs.

Although great potential for employing computer-aided processes in endoscopic surgery are being pointed out by Liedlgruber et al. [31], research concerned with classification techniques that operate on corresponding media yet is rather sparse – no matter if deep learning is applied or not. A few studies have been published by Häfner et al. within the scope of colonoscopy: they show the feasibility of automatically classifying colonic mucosa via feeding pyramidal discrete wavelet-transformed images to a k-nearest neighbors (k-NN) as well as Bayes classifier [17], develop a system for automated colon cancer detection based on the pit pattern classification (Kudo et al. [27]) in [18] and propose a novel color texture operator for pit pattern classification outperforming state-of-the-art operators in terms of compactness as well as computational speed [19]. As for CNN-based approaches, Park et al. [38] apply learning of hierarchical features on colonoscopy images for identifying polyp regions with an accuracy of 90%. Albeit in a different context, but specific to this work's target-domain – laparoscopy – Petscharnig et al. [39] continue training AlexNet (Krizhevsky et al. [25]) to be able classify shots taken from a large gynecologic video database categorized into 14 different classes in order to aid physicians in the process of surgery annotation.

Finally, surgical smoke detection is yet another area still not much researched – predominantly visual smoke recognition is addressed in non-medical settings such as identifying fire outbursts [36,47,49], utilizing classification approaches like image separation [44], optical flow computation [11,24] or pattern recognition [15,16,45]. Since smoke emergence and lighting conditions in endoscopic environments strongly differ from outdoor settings, these techniques only to some extent are applicable to the medical sector. In the field of laparoscopy, apart from a non-vision-based assessment of smoke evacuation benefits (Takahashi et al. [42]) and an US patent from the Sony Corporation vaguely describing a frame-based system using motion blur as well as pixel block analysis [9], we merely are able to discover one related study, albeit targeted towards retrieval of scenes containing smoke in contrast to their real-time detection, as is our intent: Loukas et al. [33]. They extract 76 individual shots of 26–58 frames (between 1976–4408 images) from cholecystectomy videos, calculate their space-time optical flow together with some kinematic features and employ a one-class support vector machine (OCSVM) for classification, outperforming selected wavelet-based image decomposition methods for fire surveillance [8,16,29].

3   Proposed Methodologies

Altogether, we propose three smoke classification approaches: Sect. 3.1 gives an understanding of simply inspecting an image's saturation channel in HSV color

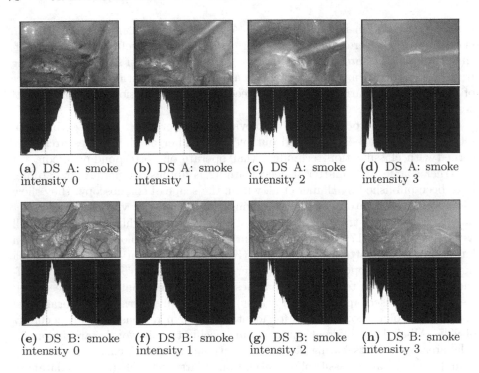

(a) DS A: smoke intensity 0   **(b)** DS A: smoke intensity 1   **(c)** DS A: smoke intensity 2   **(d)** DS A: smoke intensity 3

(e) DS B: smoke intensity 0   **(f)** DS B: smoke intensity 1   **(g)** DS B: smoke intensity 2   **(h)** DS B: smoke intensity 3

Fig. 2. Smoke development in different datasets DS A and B, including 256 bin saturation histograms. Images show various smoke intensities: none (0), weak (1), moderate (2), strong (3). Visual histogram comparison facilitated by division into four equal sectors (vertical lines).

space – a technique we call *Saturation Peak Analysis* (SPA) and Sect. 3.2 outlines the development of two GoogLeNet CNN models learned from both, full color (GLN RGB) as well as saturation only (GLN SAT) samples.

3.1   Saturation Peak Analysis (SPA)

Regions of smoke in endoscopic images tend to be grayish or rather *colorless*. Therefore, it seems appropriate to use the saturation component of the HSV color space to detect these areas, especially since the amount of smoke increases rapidly in the abdominal cavity when there is no evacuation mechanism in place. A caveat of taking such a perspective is that other colorless entities can be found during laparoscopic procedures: e.g. instruments and reflections of light hitting objects. Interferences like that can severely impact the saturation of an image, hence, naively observing this value will yield moderate classification results. Using the saturation histogram of a frame, we found in an explorative manner that by merely inspecting significant local bin maxima, i.e. *peaks* in the histogram's shape, we can determine colorlessness, compensating for insignificant non-smoke influences.

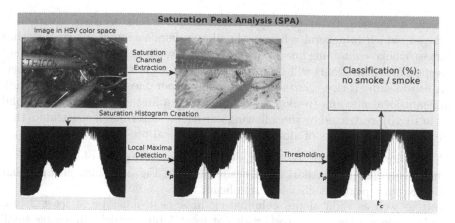

Fig. 3. SPA Classification: finding local maxima in an image's saturation histogram and classifying via thresholding. (Color figure online)

In order to illustrate the basis for our reasoning, Fig. 2 shows transitions in smoke intensities from no smoke to a very high degree of smoke together with corresponding saturation histograms for two scenes taken from different laparoscopic datasets[4]. Additionally to displaying individual pixel saturation counts via their 256 bins, the histogram images in the figure are sectioned into four equal parts indicated by three blue dashed vertical lines marking 25%, 50% and 75% portions of all bins, which helps facilitate their comparison across the portrayed smoke intensification. It can easily be discovered that the bin curves strongly correlate to the presence of smoke: for example, the depicted upper scene (Figs. 2a–d) starts out with an almost centered histogram curve (Fig. 2a) moving below the first bin quarter as smoke rises to a strong level (Fig. 2d). In contrast this development, the lower sequence's histograms (Figs. 2e–h) overall are far less saturated, predominantly gathering in between the second bin portion (Fig. 2e) but swiftly gravitating below the first one at a high level of smoke (Fig. 2h), again indicating colorlessness in similar fashion to former example. Empirical pre-study analyses on our laparoscopic video material show that these individual trends apply to the majority of images in different datasets, therefore, smoke detection using saturation histograms seemingly boils down to finding an appropriate concentration point for bin values of non-smoke samples, i.e. a classification threshold as introduced shortly, which can be used as a reference to smoke samples that generally exhibit a lower concentration point. As this is not a straightforward task, at present we incrementally select such locations and apply SPA in order to classify a single image, which is visually described in Fig. 3.

SPA analyzes a frame's saturation by converting it into the HSV color space, before isolating corresponding S-channel and creating a respective

---

[4] The image sequences show typical scenes from both of this study's custom datasets, i.e. DS A and DS B (see Sect. 4.1 for details).

intensity histogram. Using this representation, a twofold decision criterium is employed, which in general relies on the above demonstrated observation that colorless/smoke-containing images exhibit many low saturated pixels, hence their corresponding histograms will comprise higher values in their lower bins, inherently establishing a vice versa situation for the upper ones (cf. Fig. 2). In detail, significant local maxima (peaks) are computed as a first step (red vertical solid lines in Fig. 3), restricted by the following iteratively determined constraints that as well constitute results of aforementioned empirical pre-study:

- A maximum must not be found below a *peak threshold* of $t_p = 0.35 \times max\_bin\_value$ (green horizontal dashed line in Fig. 3), which ensures that a discovered peak is sufficiently significant.
- Left as well as right slopes culminating in a peak must be at least 2 bins wide rendering the peak's total width at least 5 bins, which eliminates small outliers exhibiting very similar saturation values (e.g. gray instruments).

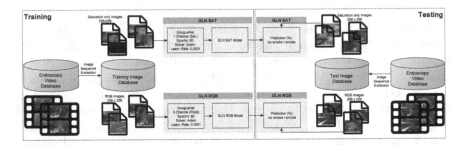

Fig. 4. CNN Training/Testing: RGB/SAT images used in GoogLeNet-based model training, evaluations via different dataset.

Finally, classification is simply based on relating the number of peaks below a *classification threshold* t_c (blue vertical dashed line in Fig. 3) to the ones above, yielding prediction confidences $pred_S$ for smoke as well as $pred_{NS}$ for non-smoke, defined by Formulas 2 and 1:

$$pred_S(pk(H)) = \frac{|\{p \mid p \in pk(H) \wedge p \leq t_c\}|}{|pk(H)|}, \tag{1}$$

$$pred_{NS}(pk(H)) = \frac{|\{p \mid p \in pk(H) \wedge p > t_c\}|}{|pk(H)|}, \tag{2}$$

where H describes a set of input histogram bin values ($|H| = 256$) and function $pk(H) \subset \mathbb{N}_0$ calculates the set of peak positions following the criteria outlined above. In case no peak is found, i.e. $pk(H) = \emptyset$, the predictions are made via finding the majority of bin's values above and below t_c, defined by Formulas 4 and 3:

$$pred_S(H) = \frac{1}{|H|} \sum_{\substack{i=0 \\ b \in H \\ i \leq t_c}} b_i, \tag{3}$$

$$pred_{NS}(H) = \frac{1}{|H|} \sum_{\substack{i=0 \\ b \in H \\ i>t_c}} b_i. \tag{4}$$

For demonstration purposes, Fig. 3 indicates a t_c of 0.50, yet for evaluation values from 0.10 up to 0.80 in 0.05 increment steps are used, which, as mentioned, currently serves the purpose of iteratively finding suitable thresholds for videos exhibiting a different color spectrum. The necessity for this decision becomes apparent when recalling pre-study discovery, formerly highlighted when discussing Fig. 2: images from separate laparoscopic datasets on average show distinguishable differences in saturation histograms. Consequently, when once again regarding the illustrated smoke intensification examples, SPA should perform best between $t_c = 0.40$ to $t_c = 0.60$ for the first and $t_c = 0.20$ to $t_c = 0.40$ for the second scene, which will be evaluated in Sect. 4.

3.2 CNN Classification

Promising image classification results achieved by using CNN architectures, most prominently LeNet [28], AlexNet [26] and GoogLeNet [41] as well as advances in applying those networks in the medical domain (see Sect. 2) inspired our impulse to employ them for our smoke classification task at hand. While utilizing deeper networks like, for instance, ResNet [20] (152 layers) may yield better results, their slower computation speed would be detrimental to our general aim – real-time smoke detection on preferably commercially available hardware. Therefore, we choose to benefit from 22-layered pre-trained CNN architecture GoogLeNet and at first pursue the most conventional strategy of simply using RGB images to continue training the network, which we further denominate GLN RGB for brevity. In order to enable a direct comparison between a trained CNN model and the SPA approach that builds on saturation analysis, we use grayscale images only depicting the saturation channel of the HSV color space for creating a classification model we accordingly label GLN SAT – a decision largely based on discovering partially very promising results when applying SPA (see Sect. 4). Figure 4 illustrates both approaches for training and classification, which are conducted via popular deep learning framework Caffe [22].

For training and validating each of the GLN architectures an 80:20 split of dataset images[5] are used with an even distribution for non-smoke/smoke samples. Exclusively in case of GLN SAT these are converted to saturation only pictures, whereas further preprocessing remained the same for both methods: resizing to GoogLeNet's intended resolution of 256×256 pixels, computation of a global image mean needed for data normalization as well as encapsulating the results within a Lightning Memory-Mapped Database (lmdb) [2].

Model training altogether takes a little over two hours for each model on a machine running Linux Mint 17.3 (64-bit) [1] with following hardware specs:

---

[5] Approximately 20 000 non-smoke/smoke images of DS A (see Sect. 4.1 for details).

Intel Core i7-3770K CPU @ 3.50GHz x 4, 16 GiB DDR3 @ 1333 MHz, Nvidia GeForce GTX 980 Ti. The Caffe solver options have iteratively been adjusted through several training attempts and finally set to: 100 Epochs – ultimately we chose Epoch 80 due to its high accuracy, stochastic optimization using Adam [23] with an initial learning rate of 0.0001.

At last, classification can be conducted merely requiring the trained model (snapshot @ 80 Epochs) in order to calculate prediction confidences for non-smoke or smoke images.

4   Experimental Results

Detailed results of all three above described methodologies and statistics are covered within this section. First, we introduce our employed datasets in Sect. 4.1. Afterwards, a closer look is taken at evaluations using test data from DS A (Subsect. 4.2), which is taken from the same source material as the GLN training data, yet it of course comprises different scenes. Afterwards, images from DS B are evaluated, which, as already mentioned, are extracted from a distinctly separate kind of source (Sect. 4.3). Finally, the overall performance of the applied methods is inspected in Subsect. 4.4.

4.1   Datasets

All our evaluations are based on two datasets: dataset A (DS A) and dataset B (DS B), described in following short paragraphs.

DS A is used for training, validation as well as testing and it consists of images taken from over eight laparoscopic surgeries in the field of gynecology. We extract different frame sequences of up to two seconds in length, amounting to about 30 000 images, half of which show non-smoke situations, the other half depicts smoke occurring in various intensities. For training and validating CNN models we use approximately 20 000 images (50% non-smoke/smoke), which leaves about 10 000 samples for evaluations.

The laparoscopic source videos for DS A show many similarities, since they are recorded under similar conditions: the same endoscope and lighting yield an analogous image color spectrum. Therefore, we added DS B, which is extracted from a laparoscopic video recorded in another location and under different circumstances. The dataset's color scheme differs in large parts from DS A, which we determined via a thorough preliminary histogram analysis and major implications, namely different optimal classification thresholds, are hinted at in Sect. 3.1, Fig. 2. Hence this dataset represents a valuable resource to solidify evaluation results. DS B consists of about 4 500 images (50% non-smoke/smoke), again taken from sequences of up to two seconds. They exclusively are used for evaluation only, which will be outlined in Sect. 4.3.

4.2 Evaluation Results - DS A

Results from evaluating DS A are illustrated in Table 1a, which lists selected classification measures for both GLN methods, as well as SPA with t_c ranging from 0.10 to 0.80 generally arranged in 0.10 increment steps except for exception $t_c = 0.45$ in order to highlight its peak performance area (see details below). Classifications in the table are conducted at confidence $c_c = 0.50$, meaning for instance that in order to correctly classify an image containing smoke, the classifier's prediction confidence for corresponding label needs to be 50% or higher (progression at different c_c values can be observed inspecting the ROC curve in Fig. 5a). For the given DS A, GLN RGB shows the best performance with 93.2% correctly classified smoke samples, i.e. very high sensitivity, and even higher specificity of 95.3%, i.e. correctly classified non-smoke samples, yielding an accuracy of 94.2%. GLN SAT achieves a slightly worse outcome but still yields a quite high accuracy of 87.0% with 82.6% sensitivity and 91.4% specificity. As for SPA, at $c_c = 50$ a threshold of $t_c = 0.40$ seems to classify similarly compared to GLN SAT, resulting in an accuracy of 85.0%, 87.7% sensitivity and 82.2% specificity. Regarding the accuracy and precision of SPA from $t_c = 0.10$ up to $t_c = 0.80$ it becomes clear that SPAs peak performance is around $t_c = 0.30$ to $t_c = 0.50$, specifically above $t_c = 0.40$, which indicates that non-smoke saturation

Table 1. Evaluation results for datasets A and B, $c_c = \mathbf{0.50}$.

(a) DS A.

Method	Accuracy	Precision	Sensitivity	Specificity	F1
GLN RGB	0.942	0.952	0.932	0.953	0.942
GLN SAT	0.870	0.906	0.826	0.914	0.864
SPA 0.10	0.536	0.891	0.081	0.990	0.149
SPA 0.20	0.674	0.968	0.360	0.988	0.525
SPA 0.30	0.770	0.928	0.585	0.955	0.718
SPA 0.40	0.850	0.831	0.877	0.822	0.854
SPA 0.45	0.820	0.752	0.956	0.685	0.842
SPA 0.50	0.738	0.659	0.986	0.491	0.790
SPA 0.60	0.557	0.530	0.999	0.115	0.693
SPA 0.70	0.506	0.503	1.000	0.013	0.670
SPA 0.80	0.500	0.500	1.000	0.000	0.667

(b) DS B.

Method	Accuracy	Precision	Sensitivity	Specificity	F1
GLN RGB	0.779	0.697	0.908	0.555	0.821
GLN SAT	0.914	0.879	0.962	0.864	0.919
SPA 0.10	0.507	0.954	0.029	0.999	0.056
SPA 0.20	0.815	0.994	0.639	0.996	0.778
SPA 0.25	0.910	0.976	0.843	0.979	0.905
SPA 0.30	0.892	0.843	0.966	0.816	0.909
SPA 0.40	0.508	0.507	1.000	0.003	0.673
SPA 0.50	0.507	0.507	1.000	0.000	0.672
SPA 0.60	0.507	0.507	1.000	0.000	0.672
SPA 0.70	0.507	0.507	1.000	0.000	0.672
SPA 0.80	0.507	0.507	1.000	0.000	0.672

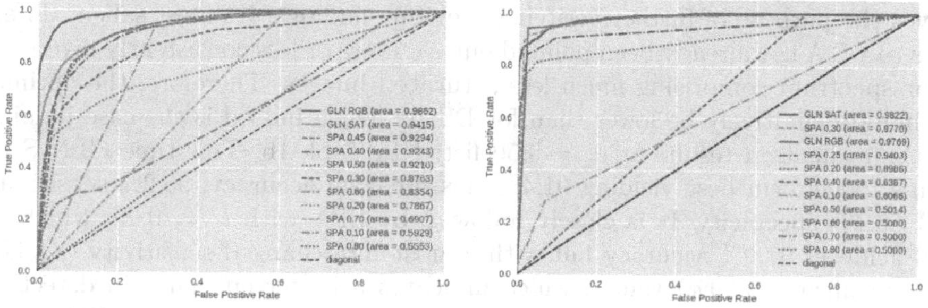

(a) DS A.

(b) DS B.

Fig. 5. ROC curve comparison for datasets A and B. (Color figure online)

histograms tend to exhibit more peaks, i.e. higher bin values, above $t_c = 0.40$ and vice-versa for smoke histograms. Figure 6 shows the most significant confusion matrices at $c_c = 0.50$, used to calculate part of the results in Table 1a.

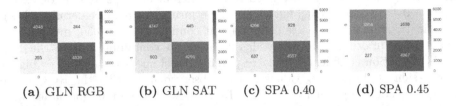

(a) GLN RGB   (b) GLN SAT   (c) SPA 0.40   (d) SPA 0.45

Fig. 6. Most significant confusion matrices for DS A (0 no smoke, 1 smoke), $c_c = \mathbf{0.50}$.

Clearly GLN RGB (Fig. 6a) with merely 599 misclassifications out of 10386 images again emphasizes the findings from above, whereas SPA 0.45 with 1865 (Fig. 6d) falsely classified samples stands out as the worst of the bunch. However, a slightly different impression can be gained when regarding a continuous c_c progression, as is depicted in Fig. 5a showing the ROC curve of the methods listed in Table 1a. Judging by the AUCs, it is evident that GLN RGB (solid blue curve) still performs best with an AUC of 0.9862, followed by GLN SAT's (solid orange curve) AUC of 0.9415. For SPA although in contrast to the above discoveries $t_c = 0.45$ (dashed green curve) seems to have an overall better performance than $t_c = 0.40$ (dashed red curve), albeit just slightly (AUC 0.9294 vs. 0.9243). Nevertheless this is interesting to see, since results for $c_c = 0.50$ seem to differ by a higher degree, which apparently is approximated as c_c progresses. SPA using other t_c values, as already pointed out, gradually perform worse up until the point of near randomness (dashed black diagonal line).

4.3   Evaluation Results - DS B

Due to the fact that DS B (around 4 000 images, 50% non-smoke/smoke), as mentioned above, has not been involved in any GLN training at all, it perfectly serves the purpose of further verifying previous findings. Its most salient difference to DS A has already been pointed out – a more or less consistently divergent color spectrum comprising much less saturated images. Therefore, the optimal t_c should definitely be lower than for DS A, which indeed is the case judging by the evaluation results at $c_c = 0.50$ listed in Table 1b. This time GLN SAT seems to perform best yielding 91.4% classification accuracy, 96.2% sensitivity and 86.4% specificity. It is closely followed by SPA with $t_c = 0.25$, which as well achieves 91.0% accuracy but with almost interchanged sensitivity (84.3%) and specificity (97.9%) values, which indicates a better efficiency in detecting non-smoke than smoke. Nevertheless, the performance sweet spot for SPA seems to lie between $t_c = 0.25$ and $t_c = 0.30$, since in the latter's outcome sensitivity (96.6%) and specificity (81.6%) are again reversed, resulting in an accuracy of

89.2%. As Fig. 7 shows, GLN RGB at $c_c = 0.50$ misclassifies a lot of non-smoke images (934 of 2098), which causes it to perform rather poorly compared to all other methods yielding unbalanced 100.0% sensitivity, 55.5% specificity and only 77.9% accuracy.

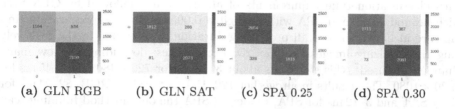

| (a) GLN RGB | (b) GLN SAT | (c) SPA 0.25 | (d) SPA 0.30 |

Fig. 7. Most significant confusion matrices for DS B (0 no smoke, 1 smoke), $c_c = \mathbf{0.50}$.

Finally, we take a look at the ROC curves from DS B's evaluations, which are depicted in Fig. 5b and again paint a slightly different picture. GLN SAT (blue solid line) with an AUC of 0.9822 still turns out to be the best classifier for DS B. SPA with $t_c = 0.30$ (orange dashed line), however, comes in second with an area of 0.9770, similarly to the DS A's evaluation, outperforming the seemingly better SPA method at $c_c = 0.50$. Surprisingly GLN RGB (green solid line) ranks third with 0.9769 only performing negligibly worse than the former method. SPA with $t_c = 0.25$ (red dashed line) classifies well yielding an AUC of 0.9403, yet performance for other SPA rapidly decreases, especially starting from $t_c = 0.40$ upwards, where many effectively yield predictions equal to a random classifier – SPA curves above $t_c = 60$ even exactly match the diagonal line.

4.4   Runtime Evaluation

Since the intent behind this work is real-time smoke detection, it is important to as well consider computational performance in addition to above assessed classification quality. Table 2 shows the average wall clock timings[6] of image *preparation, classification* and their total for both datasets' differing sample resolutions (DS A: 720×480, DS B: 1920×1080).

Table 2. Image evaluation performance avg. in DS A/B (ms).

Method	Preparation	Classification	Overall
SPA (720x480)	3.542	0.005	3.546
GLN RGB (720x480)	12.182	107.880	120.063
GLN SAT (720x480)	6.234	75.936	82.170
SPA (1920x1080)	12.487	0.006	12.493
GLN RGB (1920x1080)	45.132	105.223	150.355
GLN SAT (1920x1080)	18.847	75.307	94.154

---

[6] For the exact machine hardware specs, see Sect. 3.2.

All evaluations are implemented in Python [4] with preparation steps mostly consisting of OpenCV [3] tasks, like color conversion, image resizing and histogram extraction but as well of course a custom implementation for finding local maxima in case of SPA. Regarding the measurements for both resolutions, it becomes apparent that GLN RGB by far is the most costly of all methods with classification time requirements of about 105 ms, followed by GLN SAT with around 75 ms and SPA with negligible 0.005 ms. In case preparation timings are included, the overall processing duration worsens due to the relatively long time resizing images to 256×256 pixels takes: depending on how many channels are used[7], this step adds about 3–12 ms for 720×480 and 8–45 ms for 1920×1080. This results in altogether 120–150 ms for GLN RGB, 82–94 ms for GLN SAT and 3–12 ms for SPA, rendering SPA the only method fulfilling real-time requirements[8] on the utilized test machine.

4.5   Discussion

When surveying the entirety of outcomes, a clear trend towards GoogLeNet using colored images (GLN RGB) can be observed, since its worst performance in both datasets still is producing a ROC AUC of above 0.97. Unfortunately this as well is the most computationally expensive method, showing runtime performances of about 150 ms per HD image, which indicates merely near real-time performance. Nevertheless, since smoke development across frames does generally not change very rapidly, it would very likely be feasible to drop some frames and still achieve great results in live systems. As an alternative, GoogLeNet fed with saturation images (GLN SAT) could be used to speed up the process considerably with a performance of around 94 ms for the same type of input. This would impact classification performance but not substantially, since at worst evaluations still show an AUC of over 0.94. The only method capable of true real-time performance is saturation peak analysis (SPA) with as little as around 12 ms computation requirements and ROC curve areas of at least over 0.92, when *always* considering the best classification threshold t_c. However, SPA critically relies on finding this right t_c for every classified image, which renders the algorithm, at least in its current form, inapplicable for live smoke detection. Still, when regarding analyses conducted on DS A and B, it seems apparent that, although different surgery setups can produce contrasting distributions in saturation, equivalent ones appear to share similar values. This consideration would for example explain SPA showing optimal performance for both datasets at different threshold ranges: around $t_c = 0.40$ to $t_c = 0.50$ for DS A and $t_c = 0.20$ to $t_c = 0.30$ for DS B.

Regarding comparability with most relevant work by Loukas et al. [33] described in Sect. 2, it has to be born in mind that the authors do not target real-time smoke evacuation, as is the case in our study. Nevertheless, since our methodologies can achieve at least a near real-time classification rate, they could

---

[7] SAT channel conversion takes around 3 ms for 720×480, 10 ms for 1920×1080.

[8] For a 25 fps video real-time requirements would be: $\frac{1000}{25} = 40$ ms.

as well be utilized to annotate recorded media. In straight comparison, although outperforming selected wavelet-based outdoor smoke detection methods with an achieved ROC AUC of 0.63, their methodology seems to perform considerably worse than our proposed techniques, at least for their custom created dataset.

5   Conclusion

Targeting real-time smoke detection in endoscopic videos, we develop several image-based classification approaches, which we evaluate on two custom laparo-scopic datasets. Continued training of GoogLeNet using full color samples overall achieves the highest classification but lowest runtime performance, which could be mitigated by simply omitting frames in real-time systems. Alternatively, using saturation channel only images for GoogLeNet training still produces a high accuracy at much faster computation times, yet as well not fully capable of handling live streams. In contrast to these CNN-based methods, naive image saturation analysis shows good performance in terms of classification and run-time, however, it is currently limited to requiring information about a dataset's average saturation distribution for non-smoke images.

When addressing our general research question **Q** inquiring the feasibility of reliable smoke recognition in laparoscopic live streams, we consider the achieved classification quality to be good enough for highly accurate systems. Regarding the real-time aspect, future investigations need to be conducted, although we estimate dropping frames being a sufficient measure to compensate for slower computation speeds. Furthermore, we deem the evaluated methodologies also be applicable to general endoscopic videos, since they typically are very similar to laparoscopic recordings, where equivalent equipment is used.

In future work, we will evaluate the performance of our present method-ologies on further datasets, particularly published by others. Additionally, our promising results motivate investigating more and different CNN architectures, possibly as well many-layered architectures, despite a likely even greater impact on computation times. Finally, since saturation seems to be a good indicator for smoke, it is worthwhile to investigate histogram equalization methods for auto-matically determining good naive classification thresholds or finding alternative combinations for training CNN models.

Acknowledgements. This work was supported by Universität Klagenfurt and Lake-side Labs GmbH, Klagenfurt, Austria and funding from the European Regional Devel-opment Fund and the Carinthian Economic Promotion Fund (KWF) under grant KWF 20214 u. 3520/26336/38165.

References

1. Linux mint 17.3 "rosa" - cinnamon (64-bit) (2006). https://linuxmint.com/edition.php?id=204. Accessed 28 Mar 2017
2. Lightning memory-mapped database (2016). https://symas.com/offerings/lightning-memory-mapped-database. Accessed 28 Mar 2017

3. OpenCV library (2017). http://opencv.org/
4. Python programming language (2017). https://www.python.org/
5. Al Sahaf, O.S., Vega-Carrascal, I., Cunningham, F.O., McGrath, J.P., Bloomfield, F.J.: Chemical composition of smoke produced by high-frequency electrosurgery. Irish J. Med. Sci. **176**(3), 229–232 (2007)
6. Anthimopoulos, M., Christodoulidis, S., Ebner, L., Christe, A., Mougiakakou, S.: Lung pattern classification for interstitial lung diseases using a deep convolutional neural network. IEEE Trans. Med. Imaging **35**(5), 1207–1216 (2016). http://ieeexplore.ieee.org
7. Ball, K.: Controlling surgical smoke: A team approach. Information Booklet (2004). http://www.megadyne.com/pdf/Kay-Ball-Smoke-Booklet.pdf
8. Calderara, S., Piccinini, P., Cucchiara, R.: Vision based smoke detection system using image energy and color information. Mach. Vis. Appl. **22**(4), 705–719 (2011). http://link.springer.com/10.1007/s00138-010-0272-1
9. Chen-Rui Chou, M.C.L.: System and Method for Smoke Detection During Anatomical Surgery (2016). https://www.google.com/patents/US20160239967
10. Choi, S.H., Kwon, T.G., Chung, S.K., Kim, T.H.: Surgical smoke may be a biohazard to surgeons performing laparoscopic surgery. Surg. Endosc. Interv. Tech. **28**(8), 2374–2380 (2014)
11. Chunyu, Y., Jun, F., Jinjun, W., Yongming, Z.: Video fire smoke detection using motion and color features. Fire Technol. **46**(3), 651–663 (2010). http://link.springer.com/10.1007/s10694-009-0110-z
12. Cosmescu, I.: Automatic smoke evacuator system for a surgical laser apparatus and method therefor (1991). https://www.google.com/patents/US5199944
13. Cosmescu, I.: Automatic smoke evacuator and insufflation system for surgical procedures (2006). https://www.google.com/patents/US20070249990
14. Dobrogowski, M., Wesołowski, W., Kucharska, M., Sapota, A., Pomorski, L.: Chemical composition of surgical smoke formed in the abdominal cavity during laparoscopic cholecystectomy—assessment of the risk to the patient. Int. J. Occup. Med. Environ. Health **27**(2), 314–325 (2014). http://ijomeh.eu/Chemical-composition-of-surgical-smoke-formed-in-the-abdominal-cavity-during-laparoscopic-cholecystectomy-assessment-of-the-risk-to-the-patient,2054,0,2.html
15. Ferrari, R.J., Zhang, H., Kube, C.R.: Real-time detection of steam in video images. Pattern Recogn. **40**(3), 1148–1159 (2007)
16. Gubbi, J., Marusic, S., Palaniswami, M.: Smoke detection in video using wavelets and support vector machines. Fire Saf. J. **44**(8), 1110–1115 (2009)
17. Häfner, M., Gangl, A., Liedlgruber, M., Uhl, A., Vécsei, A., Wrba, F.: Combining Gaussian Markov random fields with the discretewavelet transform for endoscopic image classification. In: Proceedings of the DSP 2009: 16th International Conference on Digital Signal Processing (2009)
18. Hafner, M., Gangl, A., Liedlgruber, M., Uhl, A., Vecsei, A., Wrba, F.: Endoscopic image classification using edge-based features. In: 2010 20th International Conference on Pattern Recognition, pp. 2724–2727. IEEE, August 2010. http://ieeexplore.ieee.org/document/5597011/
19. Häfner, M., Liedlgruber, M., Uhl, A., Vécsei, A., Wrba, F.: Color treatment in endoscopic image classification using multi-scale local color vector patterns. Med. Image Anal. **16**(1), 75–86 (2012). http://www.sciencedirect.com/science/article/pii/S1361841511000569
20. He, K., Zhang, X., Ren, S., Sun, J.: Deep Residual Learning for Image Recognition, December 2015. http://arxiv.org/abs/1512.03385

21. Hensman, C., Baty, D., Willis, R., Cuschieri, A.: Chemical composition of smoke produced by high-frequency electrosurgery in a closed gaseous environment. Surg. Endosc. **12**, 1017 (1998). http://www.springerlink.com/index/3PDVCC89D248 BJT0.pdf

22. Jia, Y., Shelhamer, E., Donahue, J., Karayev, S., Long, J., Girshick, R., Guadarrama, S., Darrell, T.: Caffe: convolutional architecture for fast feature embedding. In: Proceedings of the 22nd ACM international conference on Multimedia, pp. 675–678. ACM (2014)

23. Kingma, D., Ba, J.: Adam: a method for stochastic optimization. arXiv preprint arXiv:1412.6980 (2014)

24. Kolesov, I., Karasev, P., Tannenbaum, A., Haber, E.: Fire and smoke detection in video with optimal mass transport based optical flow and neural networks. In: 2010 IEEE International Conference on Image Processing, pp. 761–764. IEEE, September 2010. http://ieeexplore.ieee.org/document/5652119/

25. Krizhevsky, A., Sutskever, I., Hinton, G.E.: ImageNet Classification with Deep Convolutional Neural Networks, pp. 1097–1105. Curran Associates Inc., Nevada (2012). http://papers.nips.cc/paper/4824-imagenet-classification-with-deep-con volutional-neural-networks.pdf

26. Krizhevsky, A., Sutskever, I., Hinton, G.E.: ImageNet classification with deep convolutional neural networks. In: Pereira, F., Burges, C.J.C., Bottou, L., Weinberger, K.Q. (eds.) Advances in Neural Information Processing Systems, vol. 25, pp. 1097–1105. Curran Associates, Inc., Nevada (2012). http://papers.nips.cc/paper/4824-imagenet-classification-with-deep-convolutional-neural-networks.pdf

27. Kudo, S., Hirota, S., Nakajima, T., Hosobe, S., Kusaka, H., Kobayashi, T., Himori, M., Yagyuu, A.: Colorectal tumours and pit pattern. J. Clin. Pathol. **47**(10), 880–885 (1994). http://www.ncbi.nlm.nih.gov/pubmed/7962600, http://www.pubmedcentral.nih.gov/articlerender.fcgi?artid=PMC502170

28. LeCun, Y., Bottou, L., Bengio, Y., Haffner, P.: Gradient-based learning applied to document recognition. Proc. IEEE **86**(11), 2278–2324 (1998)

29. Lee, C.Y., Lin, C.T., Hong, C.T., Su, M.T.: Smoke detection using spatial and temporal analyses. Int. J. Innov. Comput. Inf. Control **8**(7A), 4749–4770 (2012)

30. Li, Q., Cai, W., Wang, X., Zhou, Y., Feng, D.D., Chen, M.: Medical image classification with convolutional neural network. In: 2014 13th International Conference on Control Automation Robotics & Vision (ICARCV), pp. 844–848. IEEE, December 2014. http://ieeexplore.ieee.org/document/7064414/

31. Liedlgruber, M., Uhl, A.: Endoscopic image processing - an overview. In: 2009 Proceedings of 6th International Symposium on Image and Signal Processing and Analysis, pp. 707–712. IEEE, September 2009. http://ieeexplore.ieee.org/document/5297635/

32. Buffalo Filter LLC: Surgical Smoke: Education and Training (2017). http://www.buffalofilter.com/files/7914/1443/3525/Website_Training_Education_Section_10_27_2014.pdf

33. Loukas, C., Georgiou, E.: Smoke detection in endoscopic surgery videos: a first step towards retrieval of semantic events: smoke detection in endoscopic surgery videos. Int. J. Med. Robot. Comput. Assist. Surg. **11**(1), 80–94 (2015). http://doi.wiley.com/10.1002/rcs.1578

34. Mattes, D., Silajdzic, E., Mayer, M., Horn, M., Scheidbach, D., Wackernagel, W., Langmann, G., Wedrich, A.: Surgical smoke management for minimally invasive (micro)endoscopy: an experimental study. Surg. Endosc. Interv. Tech. **24**(10), 2492–2501 (2010)
35. Menes, T., Spivak, H.: Laparoscopy: searching for the proper insufflation gas. Surg. Endosc. **14**(11), 1050–1056 (2000). http://www.ncbi.nlm.nih.gov/pubmed/11116418
36. Ojo, J., Oladosu, J.: Video-based smoke detection algorithms: a chronological survey. Comput. Eng. Intell. Syst. **5**(7), 38–50 (2014)
37. Ott, D.: Smoke production and smoke reduction in endoscopic surgery: preliminary report. Endosc. Surg. Allied Technol. **1**(4), 230–232 (1993). http://www.ncbi.nlm.nih.gov/pubmed/8050026
38. Park, S.Y., Sargent, D.: Colonoscopic polyp detection using convolutional neural networks. In: International Society for Optics and Photonics, p. 978528, March 2016. http://proceedings.spiedigitallibrary.org/proceeding.aspx?doi=10.1117/12.2217148
39. Petscharnig, S., Schöffmann, K.: Deep learning for shot classification in gynecologic surgery videos. In: Amsaleg, L., Gu mundsson, G. ., Gurrin, C., Jónsson, B. ., Satoh, S. (eds.) MMM 2017. LNCS, vol. 10132, pp. 702–713. Springer, Cham (2017). doi:10.1007/978-3-319-51811-4_57
40. Sahiner, B., Chan, H.-P., Petrick, N., Wei, D., Helvie, M., Adler, D., Goodsitt, M.: Classification of mass and normal breast tissue: a convolution neural network classifier with spatial domain and texture images. IEEE Trans. Med. Imaging **15**(5), 598–610 (1996). http://ieeexplore.ieee.org/document/538937/
41. Szegedy, C., Liu, W., Jia, Y., Sermanet, P., Reed, S., Anguelov, D., Erhan, D., Vanhoucke, V., Rabinovich, A.: Going deeper with convolutions. In: Proceedings of the IEEE Conference on Computer Vision and Pattern Recognition, pp. 1–9 (2015)
42. Takahashi, H., Yamasaki, M., Hirota, M., Miyazaki, Y., Moon, J.H., Souma, Y., Mori, M., Doki, Y., Nakajima, K.: Automatic smoke evacuation in laparoscopic surgery: a simplified method for objective evaluation. Surg. Endosc. **27**(8), 2980–2987 (2013). http://link.springer.com/10.1007/s00464-013-2821-y
43. Thiébaud, H.P., Knize, M.G., Kuzmicky, P.A., Hsieh, D.P., Felton, J.S.: Airborne mutagens produced by frying beef, pork and a soy-based food. Food Chem. Toxicol. **33**(10), 821–828 (1995)
44. Tian, H., Li, W., Wang, L., Ogunbona, P.: A novel video-based smoke detection method using image separation. In: Proceedings - IEEE International Conference on Multimedia and Expo, pp. 532–537 (2012)
45. Toreyin, B.U., Dedeoglu, Y., Cetin, A.E.: Contour Based Smoke Detection in Video Using Wavelets, pp. 1–5. IEEE (2006)
46. Tsui, C., Klein, R., Garabrant, M.: Minimally invasive surgery: national trends in adoption and future directions for hospital strategy. Surg. Endosc. **27**(7), 2253–2257 (2013). http://link.springer.com/10.1007/s00464-013-2973-9
47. Wu, S., Yuan, F., Yang, Y., Fang, Z., Fang, Y.: Real-time image smoke detection using staircase searching-based dual threshold AdaBoost and dynamic analysis. IET Image Process. **9**(10), 849–856 (2015). http://digital-library.theiet.org/content/journals/10.1049/iet-ipr.2014.1032

48. Yan, Z., Zhan, Y., Peng, Z., Liao, S., Shinagawa, Y., Zhang, S., Metaxas, D.N., Zhou, X.S.: Multi-Instance deep learning: discover discriminative local anatomies for bodypart recognition. IEEE Trans. Med. Imaging **35**(5), 1332–1343 (2016). http://ieeexplore.ieee.org/document/7398101/
49. Yuan, F.: Video-based smoke detection with histogram sequence of LBP and LBPV pyramids. Fire Saf. J. **46**(3), 132–139 (2011)

6th International Workshop on Clinical Image-Based Procedures, CLIP 2017

Fully Automatic Detection of Distal Radius Fractures from Posteroanterior and Lateral Radiographs

Raja Ebsim[1(✉)], Jawad Naqvi[2], and Tim Cootes[1]

[1] The University of Manchester, Manchester, UK
{raja.ebsim,tim.cootes}@manchester.ac.uk
[2] Health Education North West School of Radiology, Manchester, UK
naqvi.jawad@gmail.com

Abstract. We describe a fully-automated system for analysing X-rays of the wrist to identify possible fractures. Fractures of the distal radius in the wrist are estimated to be about 18% of the fractures seen in adults and 25% of those seen in children. Unfortunately such fractures are amongst the most frequently missed by doctors in Emergency Departments (EDs). A system which can identify suspicious areas could reduce the number of misdiagnoses. We automatically locate the outline of the radius in both posteroanterior (PA) and lateral (LAT) radiographs, then use shape and texture features to classify abnormalities. We show for the first time that fractures can be better identified in the lateral view, and that combining information from both views leads to an overall improvement in performance.

Keywords: Image analysis · Image interpretation and understanding · X-ray fracture detection · Wrist fractures · Radius fractures · Machine learning

1 Introduction

Fractures of the wrist are usually identified in Emergency Departments by doctors examining lateral (LAT) and posterioanterior (PA) radiographs (Fig. 1). Unfortunately missing such fractures is one of the most common diagnostic errors in EDs, leading to delayed treatment and more suffering for the patient [7,14,18]. This is mainly because the majority of patients attending EDs are seen by junior doctors [8,13]. This problem is widely acknowledged, so in many hospitals X-rays are reviewed by an expert radiologist at a later date - however this can lead to significant delays on missed fractures which can have an impact on the eventual outcome. To address this we are developing a system which can automatically analyse radiographs of the wrist in order to identify abnormalities and thus prompt clinicians, hopefully reducing the number of errors.

In this paper we describe a fully-automated system for detecting radius fractures in PA and LAT radiographs. For each view, a global search [11] is performed

© Springer International Publishing AG 2017
M.J. Cardoso et al. (Eds.): CARE/CLIP 2017, LNCS 10550, pp. 91–98, 2017.
DOI: 10.1007/978-3-319-67543-5_8

for finding the approximate position of the radius. The detailed outline of the bone is then located using a Random Forest Regression Voting Constrained Local Model (RFCLM) [10]. We use features derived from the shape and texture to train random forest classifiers on the task of detecting fractures. Features from both views are combined for better performance.

This paper is the first to show an automatic system for identifying fractures from lateral view radiographs of the wrist. We show that better performance can be achieved from this view than the PA view, and that further improvement can be obtained by combining results from both views.

2   Background

Distal radius fractures have been on increase in all age groups [15]. They alone constitute around 18% of the fractures seen in EDs in adults [4,6] and 25% of the fractures seen in children [6].

Previous work on detecting fractures in X-rays has been done on a variety of anatomical regions, including arm fractures [19], femur fractures [1,9,12,17,20], and vertebral endplates [16]. Cao *et al.* [2] used stacked random forests to fuse different feature representations to identify fractures in a range of anatomical regions. They achieved a sensitivity of 81% and precision of 25%. All reported work on automatical analysis of wrist fractures that we are aware of [5,9,12] uses only the PA view. In each case some form of shape model is used to locate the outline of the bones, then texture (and possibly shape) features are used to train a classifier to distinguish healthy from fractured bones.

[9,12] use both active shape models and active appearance models [3] to locate the approximate contour of the radius. They extract various texture features (Gabor, Markov Random Field, and gradient intensity) and classify with a Support Vector Machine SVM. They achieved encouraging performance (accuracy $\approx$ sensitivity $\approx$ 96%) but were working on a rather small dataset with only 23 fractured examples in their test set. In previous work [5] we used RFCLMs to segment both the radius and ulna in PA views and trained random forest classifiers on statistical shape parameters and eigen-mode texture features. The automatic system [5] achieved a performance of 88.6% (Area under Receiver Operating Characteristic Curve AUC) on data set of 409 radiographs including 199 fractures. The system we describe below is for the radius in both PA and LAT views achieving better performance and is tested on a data set about twice the size.

3   Method

The outline of the radius was manually annotated with 48 points in the PA view and with 64 points in the LAT View (Fig. 1). For each view, a statistical shape model and an RFCLM [10] object detection model were built from the corresponding manual annotations. The models then used to segment the bone on new radiographs automatically.

3.1 Modeling and Matching

Building Models for Shape and Texture. The outline of the radius is modeled by a linear statistical shape model [3].

Each training image is annotated with n feature points, (x_i, y_i). A $2n$-D vector $\mathbf{x} = (x_1, ..., x_n, y_1, ..., y_n)^T$ represents all the points.

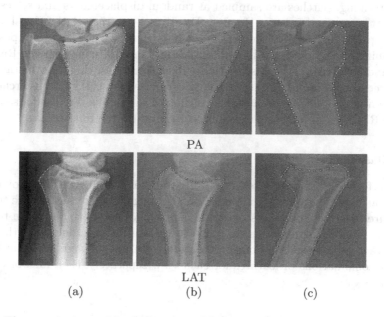

PA

LAT

(a)   (b)   (c)

Fig. 1. The annotations of both views on (a) a normal radius, (b) a radius with a subtle fracture, and (c) with an obvious fracture. The two red points, appearing on each view, are the anatomical points found by the global searcher for that view. (Color figure online)

Shapes are modelled using

$$\mathbf{x} = T(\bar{\mathbf{x}} + \mathbf{Pb} : \theta) \tag{1}$$

where $\bar{\mathbf{x}}$ is the mean shape, $\mathbf{P}$ is the set of the eigenvectors corresponding to the t highest eignvalues of the covariance matrix, $\mathbf{b}$ is the vector of shape parameters and $T(. : \theta)$ applies a similarity transformation with parameters θ. The first three modes of the built shape models are shown in Fig. 2. Similarly, statistical texture models [3] are built by applying PCA to vectors of normalised intensity $(\mathbf{g})$ sampled from the regions defined by the points of the shape model.

$$\mathbf{g} \approx \bar{\mathbf{g}} + \mathbf{P}_g \mathbf{b}_g \tag{2}$$

After fitting the model to a new radiograph, shape parameters $\mathbf{b}$ (in Eq. 1) and the texture parameters $\mathbf{b}_g$ (in Eq. 2) are used as features on which classifiers are trained to distinguish between normal and fractured bones.

Matching Shape Models to New Radiographs. We use a technique similar to that described by Lindner *et al.* [11] to locate the outline of the targeted bone in each view separately. A single global model per view is trained to initially find approximate position of a box containing two anatomical landmarks (i.e. the red points in Fig. 1). As in [11] a random forest regressor with Hough voting is trained to find the displacement between the center of a patch and the object center. During training, patches are sampled at random displacements and scales from the object center and fed to a Random Forest to learn the relationship between an image patch and the displacement of the patch centre from the target position. By scanning a new image at different scales and orientations with the Random Forest and collecting the votes, the most likely center, scale and orientation of the object can be found. The two points estimated by the global searcher are used to initialise a local search for the outline of the radius. We used a sequence of three RFCLMs of increasing resolution to produce the final result.

3.2   Classification

After performing the full automatic search so that radius outline points are located on all radiographs, Random Forest classifiers (100 trees each) are trained on features derived from the shape (the shape parameters, $\mathbf{b}$) and the texture (the texture model parameters, $\mathbf{b}_g$) for the task of fracture detection (i.e. normal or fractured). A series of cross validation experiments were performed with different combinations of features for each view separately, then for both views together.

4   Experiments

Data. The experiments were carried out on a dataset containing both views for 787 adult patients (378 of whom had fractures) from two local EDs gathered and anonymised by a clinician.

Automatic Annotation. In order to generate the automatic annotation for the whole dataset, we divided PA radiographs into two subsets, training models on one subset and applying them to the second. Four subsets were needed to successfully learn representative models for the LAT view. That is because of the overlap between the two bones, (i.e. radius and ulna) on lateral view can take various orientations due to different acceptable positioning in practice [6]. This is not the case for PA view as the two bones appear side by side. Figure 3 shows some examples from our LAT dataset.

The accuracy of the segmentation is calculated as the percentage of mean point-to-curve distance [11] to a reference width, and converted to mm by assuming a mean reference width of 25 mm for the radius in the PA view and 20 mm in the LAT view. The reference width of a view is the distance between the two reference points for that view (see Fig. 1(a)).

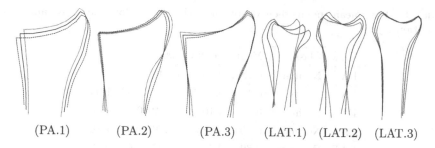

(PA.1)   (PA.2)   (PA.3)   (LAT.1)   (LAT.2)   (LAT.3)

Fig. 2. The first three modes of the shape models of the radius.

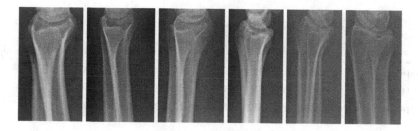

Fig. 3. Different relative radius-ulna positions appearing in lateral radiographs.

The results in Table 1 show the ability of the models to successfully segment the targeted structure even when fractured. The mean error was less than 1.4 mm for more than 95% of the radiographs in the LAT view and less than 0.6 mm for 95% of radiographs in the PA view. The PA error was less that reported in [5] (0.61 mm vs 0.78 mm for the 95%-ile, though our dataset is twice the size). The table also breaks down the results by class and shows that although in the PA view there is almost no difference in accuracy between fractured and normal cases, in the LAT view errors are roughly 50% larger. However overall the system can successfully capture a good approximation to both the normal and fractured shapes.

Classification. For each view we performed 5-fold cross validation experiments with Random Forest classifiers using 100 trees (repeated three times) on: (i) shape parameters only, (ii) texture parameters only, and (iii) the concatenation of shape and texture parameters. The results obtained from the PA view, shown in Table 2, reflects the small difference between the manual and automatic annotation. The performance of the automated system improves slightly on that described in [5] (though that was on a smaller dataset).

Table 3 shows the classification results for the LAT view. Note that classifying using the shape alone gives significantly better performance than that from the PA view. Adding the texture information makes only a small improvement (in the manual case) and slightly degrades performance of the fully automated system. The difference in performance for shape between manual and automatic

Table 1. The mean point-to-curve distance in (mm) for the fully automatic annotations.

View	Class	Mean	Median	90%	95%	99%
PA	Normal	0.18	0.10	0.40	0.50	1.08
PA	Fractured	0.18	0.11	0.47	0.63	1.04
PA	Both	0.18	0.10	0.42	0.61	1.06
LAT	Normal	0.40	0.28	0.76	0.94	1.86
LAT	Fractured	0.62	0.44	1.27	1.62	2.83
LAT	Both	0.50	0.32	1.01	1.37	2.34

Table 2. AUC for classification based on PA view.

PA view	Manual	Fully automated	Automated result from [5]
Shape	0.847 ± 0.004	0.826 ± 0.002	0.816 ± 0.007
Texture	0.896 ± 0.005	0.891 ± 0.001	**0.881 ± 0.004**
Shape & Texture	**0.898 ± 0.002**	**0.897 ± 0.002**	0.868 ± 0.002

results suggests that classification performance can be improved by improving the accuracy of the search (perhaps by increasing the size of the training set).

Table 3. AUC for classification based on lateral view.

LAT view	Manual	Fully automated
Shape	0.933 ± 0.001	**0.905 ± 0.003**
Texture	0.894 ± 0.002	0.878 ± 0.002
Shape & Texture	**0.937 ± 0.001**	0.899 ± 0.001

Combining information from both views results in the best classification performance in both manual and automatic cases. See Table 4. Figure 4 shows the ROC curves for the best results.

Table 4. AUC for classification based on features from both views.

PA & LAT views	Manual	Fully automated
Shape	0.933 ± 0.001	0.913 ± 0.003
Texture	0.918 ± 0.002	0.890 ± 0.006
Shape & Texture	**0.942 ± 0.002**	**0.914 ± 0.004**

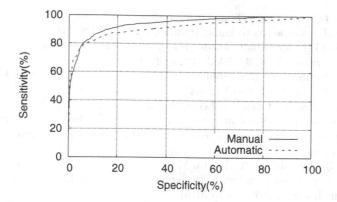

Fig. 4. The ROC curves corresponding to classification based on combining shape and texture features from both PA and LAT views for: (i) manual annotation, and (ii) automatic annotation.

5 Conclusions

This paper presents a system that automatically locates the outline of radius in both posteroanterior and lateral radiographs and extracts discriminative features for fracture detection. In future work, we will extend our current work to generate automatic description of the found fracture (i.e. fracture classification), and will explore learning alternative texture features. Our long term goal is to build a system which works well enough to help clinicians in EDs make more reliable decisions.

Acknowledgment. The research leading to these results has received funding from Libyan Ministry of Higher Education and Research. The authors would like to thank Dr Jonathan Harris, Dr Matthew Davenport, and Dr Martin Smith for their collaboration to set up the project.

References

1. Bayram, F., Çakirolu, M.: DIFFRACT: diaphyseal femur fracture classifier system. Biocybern. Biomed. Eng. **36**(1), 157–171 (2016)
2. Cao, Y., Wang, H., Moradi, M., Prasanna, P., Syeda-Mahmood, T.F.: Fracture detection in x-ray images through stacked random forests feature fusion. In: International Symposium on Biomedical Imaging (ISBI 2015), pp. 801–805, April 2015
3. Cootes, T.F., Edwards, G.J., Taylor, C.J.: Active appearance models. IEEE Trans. Pattern Anal. Mach. Intell. **23**(6), 681–685 (2001)
4. Court-Brown, C.M., Caesar, B.: Epidemiology of adult fractures: a review. Injury **37**, 691–697 (2006)
5. Ebsim, R., Naqvi, J., Cootes, T.: Detection of wrist fractures in X-Ray images. In: Shekhar, R., et al. (eds.) CLIP 2016. LNCS, vol. 9958, pp. 1–8. Springer, Cham (2016). doi:10.1007/978-3-319-46472-5_1

6. Goldfarb, C.A., Yin, Y., Gilula, L.A., Fisher, A.J., Boyer, M.I.: Wrist fractures: what the clinician wants to know. Radiology **219**, 11–28 (2001)
7. Guly, H.R.: Injuries initially misdiagnosed as sprained wrist (beware the sprained wrist). Emergency Med. J. (EMJ) **19**, 41 (2002)
8. Lee, C., Bleetman, A.: Commonly missed injuries in the accident and emergency department. Trauma **6**, 41–51 (2004)
9. Lim, S.E., Xing, Y., Chen, Y., Leow, W.K., Howe, T.S., Png, M.A.: Detection of femur and radius fractures in x-ray images. In: Proceedings of 2nd International Conference on Advances in Medical Signal and Information Processing, vol. 1, pp. 249–256 (2004)
10. Lindner, C., Bromiley, P.A., Ionita, M.C., Cootes, T.: Robust and accurate shape model matching using random forest regression-voting. IEEE Trans. Pattern Anal. Mach. Intell. **37**(9), 1862–1874 (2015)
11. Lindner, C., Thiagarajah, S., Wilkinson, J.M., Consortium, T., Wallis, G.A., Cootes, T.F.: Fully automatic segmentation of the proximal femur using random forest regression voting. Med. Image Anal. **32**(8), 1462–1472 (2013)
12. Lum, V.L.F., Leow, W.K., Chen, Y., Howe, T.S., Png, M.A.: Combining classifiers for bone fracture detection in X-ray images, vol. 1, pp. I-1149–1152 (2005)
13. McLauchlan, C.A., Jones, K., Guly, H.R.: Interpretation of trauma radiographs by junior doctors in accident and emergency departments: a cause for concern? J. Accid. Emerg. Med. **14**(5), 295–298 (1997)
14. Petinaux, B., Bhat, R., Boniface, K., Aristizabal, J.: Accuracy of radiographic readings in the emergency department. Am. J. Emerg. Med. **29**, 18–25 (2011)
15. Porrino, J.A., Maloney, E., Scherer, K., Mulcahy, H., Ha, A.S., Allan, C.: Fracture of the distal radius: epidemiology and premanagement radiographic characterization. Am. J. Roentgenol. (AJR) **203**, 551–559 (2014)
16. Roberts, M.G., Oh, T., Pacheco, E.M.B., Mohankumar, R., Cootes, T.F., Adams, J.E.: Semi-automatic determination of detailed vertebral shape from lumbar radiographs using active appearance models. Osteoporos. Int. **23**(2), 655–664 (2012)
17. Tian, T.P., Chen, Y., Leow, W.K., Hsu, W., Howe, T.S., Png, M.A.: Computing neck-shaft angle of femur for X-Ray fracture detection. In: Petkov, N., Westenberg, M.A. (eds.) CAIP 2003. LNCS, vol. 2756, pp. 82–89. Springer, Heidelberg (2003). doi:10.1007/978-3-540-45179-2_11
18. Wei, C.-J., Tsai, W.-C., Tiu, C.-M., Wu, H.-T., Chiou, H.-J., Chang, C.-Y.: Systematic analysis of missed extremity fractures in emergency radiology. Acta Radiologica **47**, 710 (2006)
19. Jia, Y.: Active contour model with shape constraints for bone fracture detection. In: International Conference on Computer Graphics, Imaging and Visualisation (CGIV 2006), vol. 3, pp. 90–95 (2006)
20. Yap, D.W.H., Chen, Y., Leow, W.K., Howe, T.S., Png, M.A.: Detecting femur fractures by texture analysis of trabeculae. In: Proceedings - International Conference on Pattern Recognition vol. 3, pp. 730–733 (2004)

Automated Characterization of Pyelocalyceal Anatomy Using CT Urograms to Aid in Management of Kidney Stones

Yuankai Huo[1], Vaughn Braxton[2], S. Duke Herrell[2],
Bennett Landman[1], and Smita De[2(✉)]

[1] Vanderbilt University, Nashville, TN, USA
[2] Vanderbilt University Medical Center, Nashville, TN, USA
smita.de@vanderbilt.edu

Abstract. Nephrolithiasis is a costly and prevalent disease that is associated with significant morbidity including pain, infection, and kidney injury. While surgical treatment of kidney stones is generally based on the size and quality of the stones, studies have suggested that specific characteristics of the pyelocalyceal anatomy (i.e. urinary drainage system), such as the infundibulopelvic angle (IPA), can influence the success rate of various treatment modalities. However, the traditional methods of quantifying such anatomic features have typically relied on manual measurements using 2-dimensional (2D) images of a 3-dimensional (3D) system, which can be cumbersome and potentially inaccurate. In this paper, we propose a novel algorithm that automatically identifies and isolates the 3D volume and central frame of the urinary drainage system from computerized tomography (CT) Urograms, which then allows for 3D characterization of the pyelocalyceal anatomy. First, the kidney and pyelocalyceal system were segmented from adjacent soft tissues using an automated algorithm. A centerline tree structure was then generated from the segmented pyelocalyceal anatomy. Finally, the IPA was measured using the derived reconstructions and tree structure. 8 of 11 pyelocalyceal systems were successfully segmented and used to measure the IPA, suggesting that it is technically feasible to use our algorithm to automatically segment the pyelocalyceal anatomy from target images and determine its 3D central frame for anatomic characterization. To the best of our knowledge, this is the first method that allows for an automated characterization of the isolated 3D pyelocalyceal structure from CT images.

Keywords: Pyelocalyceal anatomy · Kidney stones · Automated segmentation

1 Introduction

The prevalence of kidney stone disease, or nephrolithiasis, has been rising over the last several decades and now affects approximately 1 in 11 individuals in the United States [1]. Most stones that do not spontaneously pass will require surgical treatment with ureteroscopy (retrograde endoscopy through the urethra and bladder), extracorporeal shock wave lithotripsy (stones fragmentation using noninvasive shock waves), percutaneous lithotripsy

© Springer International Publishing AG 2017
M.J. Cardoso et al. (Eds.): CARE/CLIP 2017, LNCS 10550, pp. 99–107, 2017.
DOI: 10.1007/978-3-319-67543-5_9

(endoscopy through 1 cm direct puncture into the kidney), or very rarely laparoscopic or open surgery. An efficient and effective choice of surgical approach is critical given the significant morbidity due to kidney stones, including pain, infection, and renal insufficiency, as well as associated costs, which were estimated to be over $5 billion in 2000 [2]. Currently, more than 40% of patients may not be stone free after surgery [3].

In determining an optimal surgical approach, it is essential to consider anatomic factors and stone features as these affect treatment success rates [4, 5]. However, prior research correlating specific characteristics of the pyelocalyceal anatomy (kidney drainage or urinary collecting system where stones grow), such as the IPA (angle representing the lower pole (i.e. most inferior portion of the drainage system where stones can settle)) and stone-free rates after surgery has often relied on manual measurements of 2D imaging modalities, such as fluoroscopy and intravenous pyelograms, to characterize the 3D urinary collecting system. Data from such studies are conflicting, which may in part be due to the crudeness of the 2D approximations [4, 6]. For example, the range of IPAs in patients using 2D intravenous urograms are not consistent with those measured from 3D resin casts of cadaver kidneys [7, 8]. Furthermore, many of the studies were performed using images taken during surgery, meaning the images were not available pre-operatively to actually aid in treatment planning.

The above indicate a strong need and opportunity for improvement in image-based patient-specific preoperative planning and counseling in the management of stone disease. The high prevalence of CT as a clinical tool provides an ideal avenue to develop algorithms for patient-specific computer-aided treatment guidance. In addition, this type of data at a population level will be highly valuable in the development of novel devices for kidney stone surgery and more general characterization of anatomy.

In this feasibility study, we aimed to automatically segment and isolate the 3D structure of the renal collecting system anatomy in normal CT Urograms that could then be used to measure the IPA, a key feature previously identified as potentially correlating with operative accessibility and thus, success of a given surgical approach.

2   Methods

2.1   Patient Selection and Imaging

The Institutional Review Board approved this study with a waiver of informed consent. Electronic medical records were used to randomly identify patients who had a CT Urogram for evaluation of hematuria (blood in the urine) [9]. Exclusion criteria included any treated or untreated kidney pathology including tumors, presence of kidney stones, anatomic variants, and chronic renal insufficiency as this affects the rate of contrast excretion. Images were manually reviewed to confirm good image quality. All excretory phase sequences (Fig. 1 demonstrates difference between a non-contrast and excretory phase image) in this study were performed in the prone position at an 8 min delay per institutional protocol with 3 mm axial reconstructions.

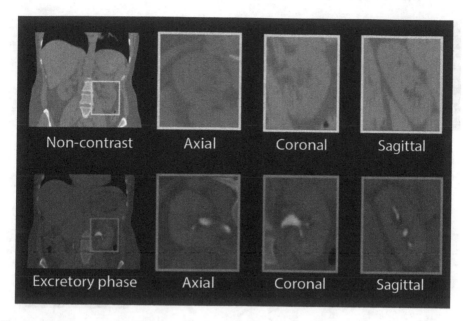

Fig. 1. Top: Non-contrast CT with cropped images of the kidney in which pyelocalyceal system is not visualized. Bottom: Excretory phase of CT Urogram with cropped images of kidney and pyelocalyceal anatomy illuminated during excretion of contrast by the kidneys.

2.2 Automated Localization and Segmentation of Whole Kidney

Figure 2 demonstrates the workflow of the proposed algorithm. A SIMPLE context learning-based multi-atlas segmentation framework [10] was used to achieve whole kidney segmentation. To achieve the SIMPLE framework, 30 pairs of atlases (anatomical CT scans and corresponding labels) were obtained from MICCAI 2015 MeDiCAL challenges (https://www.synapse.org/#!Synapse:syn3193805/wiki/89480). Two sets of cropped atlases were then formed based on kidney locations (30 pairs each for the left and right kidneys). The atlases were manually cropped by an experienced rater using MIPAV software [11]. Next, the left and right kidneys in target CT Urogram images were automatically localized and cropped using a random forest based localization method [12]. The previously cropped atlases were then registered to the cropped target CT Urogram images using affine and non-rigid registrations by NiftyReg [13]. A SIMPLE based context learning procedure was performed to select the best 10 registered atlases for each target kidney [14]. Finally, the left and right kidney segmentations from the target images were separately derived by performing a joint label fusion (JLF) [15] on the selected atlases.

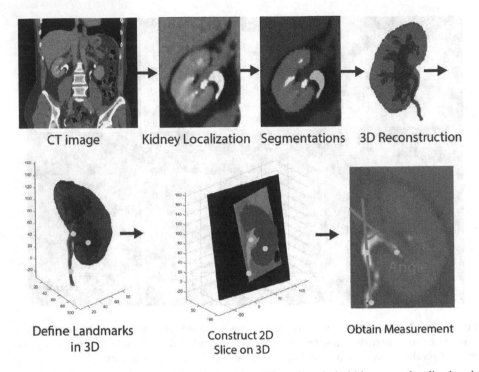

Fig. 2. The workflow of the proposed algorithm. First, the whole kidney was localized and segmented using multi-atlas segmentation. The pyelocalyceal structure was then segmented using a Gaussian Mixture Model and the tree structure was subsequently derived. Key landmarks (yellow dots) were identified from the 3D reconstruction and tree structure to construct an oblique 4 mm thick plane from which the IPA was measured. (Color figure online)

2.3 Automated Segmentation of Pyelocalyceal Anatomy and Validation

Once the kidneys were cropped and segmented from the original excretory phase images, a Gaussian mixture model (GMM) was used to segment the pyelocalyceal anatomy within the kidneys. Empirically, a threshold above 100 Hounsfield Unit (HU) was applied to exclude tissues surrounding the kidney. The GMM with three components was then employed on the histogram of remaining intensities. The two components (from three total) with higher mean HU score were clustered and identified to be the pyelocalyceal anatomy segmentation. The component with smallest mean HU score represented residual kidney organ tissue not completed removed in the initial thresholding step. Finally, a 3D tree structure (center line) was derived from the pyelocalyceal anatomy segmentation using the method described in [16]. Briefly, the method calculated the 3D axis skeleton of the 3D binary volume using a parallel thinning algorithm based on an Euler table.

All pyelocalyceal segmentations were qualitatively evaluated by a radiologist and rated as having excellent, acceptable, or poor accuracy. A random subset of the kidneys that resulted in excellent or acceptable segmentations were then manually segmented by a radiologist and the Dice coefficient was calculated.

2.4 Measurement of Infundibulopelvic Angle in 2D and 3D Images

The previously described Elbahnasy method for IPA measurement in 2D images was modified to allow for IPA measurement using 3D images and the above derived 3D tree structure [17]. Key landmarks corresponding to those in the Elbahnasy method were manually identified by a Urologist in 3D slicer software (https://www.slicer.org) using the kidney segmentation, pyelocalyceal anatomy and tree structure derived from above automated algorithm. The landmarks based on the Elbahnasy method were as follows: (1) the center point of the proximal ureter at the lowest plane of the kidney, (2) the center point of the renal pelvis along medial margin of kidney, (3) a point in the inferior branch

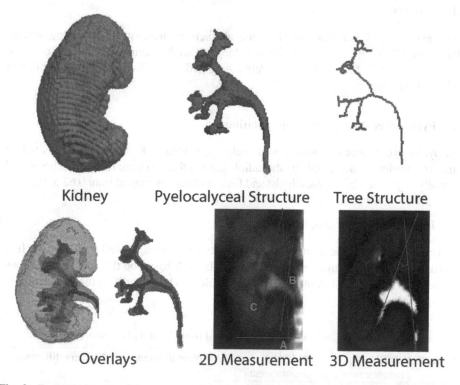

Fig. 3. Example results of the segmentation and angle measurements for a single kidney. Top row: 3D reconstruction of the kidney, 3D reconstruction of the pyelocalyceal structure, tree structure. Bottom row: Overlays of reconstructions and tree structure, traditional 2D measurement [14] of IPA (red lines) using an averaged (i.e. flattened) pseudo-2D image generated from CT images to simulate IV pyelogram IPA measurement (horizontal blue line indicates lowest plane of the kidney, sloped vertical blue line indicates medial margin of kidney, (A) center of ureter at lower margin of kidney, (B) center of renal pelvis at medial margin, (C) center line through lower pole branch), and the 3D IPA measurement (red lines) using described method. (Color figure online)

of the kidney drainage system (i.e. lower pole). The three points were used to create a unique 4 mm thick slice from the 3D volume, and the IPA was measured as the angle between the line connecting points (1) and (2), and the center line through the lowest branch of the kidney drainage system (Fig. 2).

As a comparison, 2D measurements of the IPA were performed on the cropped kidney from an averaged CT image in the coronal direction. This traditional 2D measurement was obtained by estimating the center point (A) of the proximal ureter at the lowest plane of the kidney, estimating the center point (B) of the renal pelvis along medial margin of kidney, approximating the center line (C) through the lower pole branch, and measuring the angle between line C and a line connecting A and B (Fig. 3).

3   Results

3.1   Patients

After exclusion of patients with imaging artifacts or inadequate collecting system distension, CT images of 11 individual kidneys from 8 patients were identified to be appropriate for this feasibility study. Patients ranged in age from 41–80 years old and all had normal kidney function.

3.2   Pyelocalyceal Anatomy Segmentation

The pyelocalyceal anatomy was appropriately segmented in 8 of the 11 kidneys with a rating of excellent or acceptable by the radiologist. Of these, 6 were randomly chosen and manually segmented by the radiologist and Dice coefficients ranged from 0.62 to 0.88.

3.3   Infundibulopelvic Angle

Figure 3 demonstrates the segmentation results, tree structure, as well as 2D and 3D IPA measurements from a single example kidney. The IPA based on the 3D segmentations and tree structures ranged from 14.6° to 81.5° while IPA based on 2D reformatted images

Table 1. Infundibulopelvic angles obtained from 2D and 3D measurements

Kidney#	2D IPA measurement (°)	3D IPA measurement (°)	Absolute difference (°)	Percent difference
1	19.2	23.7	4.5	18.99%
2	16.5	21.9	5.4	24.66%
3	66.9	70.1	3.2	4.57%
4	34.2	48.6	14.4	29.63%
5	57.4	60	2.6	4.33%
6	9.4	14.6	5.2	35.63%
7	16.3	19.7	3.4	17.26%
8	88.3	81.5	6.8	8.34%

ranged from 9.4° to 88.3° (Table 1). Comparisons between the angles based on the 2D and 3D methods demonstrated differences up to 35.6%.

4 Discussion

Kidney stone disease is a chronic condition that often requires many surgeries over a patient's lifetime. Each surgery is associated with risks and residual stones can have severe consequences so appropriate pre-operative evaluation and intervention are critical [18]. In addition to stone-free rates after surgery, anatomic variation may play a role in stone formation and burden of disease [6]. Thus, accurate characterization of patient anatomy can have both immediate and long-term effects with respect to surgical planning as well as lifelong management, such as the interval between imaging studies.

Augmentation of currently widely available CT Urography with powerful post-processing tools such as 3D modeling and characterization algorithms may aid in advancing patient-tailored medicine in urologic disease. While there is prior work on automated detection of kidney stones and kidney tumors [19, 20] from CT images, this is the first method known to the authors for automated isolation and characterization of the 3D pyelocalyceal frame. There have been some efforts to perform automated identification and segmentation of the pyelocalyceal anatomy using magnetic resonance imaging (MRI). A mean Dice coefficient of 0.72 [21] has been reported, which is within the range achieved in this study, but anatomic characterization was not performed and furthermore, MRIs do not provide adequate visualization of kidney stones and thus are not used for stone patients. The results presented here demonstrate that the proposed algorithm is technically feasible with CT imaging and Dice coefficient calculations indicate that the automated segmentation results compare favorably with manual segmentations for the given geometry.

With respect to the IPA, the relative difference in the measured IPA between the 2D and 3D techniques was noted to be up to 35%. As previously mentioned, prior studies have indicated that anatomic variation may be critical to predicting surgical success, but the data on IPA and other anatomic parameters are inconsistent [4]. As this preliminary data suggests, the discrepancies may be partially attributed to the lower anatomic fidelity of the traditionally utilized 2D images, and the advantages of using 3D techniques are a focus of our future studies. An inherent limitation of such automated algorithms is that the result will only be as reliable as the initial imaging, and imaging quality of CT urograms can be dependent on multiple factors such as kidney function and level of hydration. We aim to further automate our algorithm, assess additional anatomic variables, both novel and previously described, and then correlate these more accurate 3D-based measurements with stone-free rates after stone surgery. Outcomes from such studies may provide valuable tools for patient-specific stone management.

Acknowledgements. This research was supported by the Vanderbilt Institute for Surgery and Engineering (VISE) Fellowship (De), NSF CAREER 1452485 (Landman), NIH grant 5R21EY024036 (Landman), NIH grant 1R21NS064534 (Landman), and NIH grant 1R03EB012461 (Landman). This study was supported in part by VISE/VICTR VR3029 and the National Center for Research Resources, Grant UL1 RR024975-01, and is now the National

Center for Advancing Translational Sciences, Grant 2 UL1 TR000445-06. The project was also supported in part by using the resources of the Advanced Computing Center for Research and Education (ACCRE) at Vanderbilt University, Nashville, TN. The content is solely the responsibility of the authors and does not necessarily represent the official views of the NIH. The authors have no conflict of interest to declare.

References

1. Scales, C.D.J., Smith, A.C., Hanley, J.M., Saigal, C.S.: Prevalence of kidney stones in the United States. Eur. Urol. **62**, 160–165 (2012)
2. Saigal, C.S., Joyce, G., Timilsina, A.R.: Direct and indirect costs of nephrolithiasis in an employed population: opportunity for disease management? Kidney Int. **68**, 1808–1814 (2005)
3. Ghani, K.R., Wolf, J.S.: What is the stone-free rate following flexible ureteroscopy for kidney stones? Nat. Rev. Urol. **12**, 281–288 (2015)
4. Danuser, H., Müller, R., Descoeudres, B., Dobry, E., Studer, U.E.: Extracorporeal shock wave lithotripsy of lower calyx calculi: how much is treatment outcome influenced by the anatomy of the collecting system? Eur. Urol. **52**, 539–546 (2007)
5. Geavlete, P., Multescu, R., Geavlete, B.: Influence of pyelocaliceal anatomy on the success of flexible ureteroscopic approach. J. Endourol. **22**, 2235–2239 (2008)
6. Zomorrodi, A., Buhluli, A., Fathi, S.: Anatomy of the collecting system of lower pole of the kidney in patients with a single renal stone: a comparative study with individuals with normal kidneys. Saudi J. Kidney Dis. Transpl. **21**, 666–672 (2010)
7. Marroig, B., Favorito, L.A., Fortes, M.A., Sampaio, F.J.B.: Lower pole anatomy and mid-renal-zone classification applied to flexible ureteroscopy: experimental study using human three-dimensional endocasts. Surg. Radiol. Anat. **37**, 1243–1249 (2015)
8. Gozen, A.S., Kilic, A.S., Aktoz, T., Akdere, H.: Renal anatomical factors for the lower calyceal stone formation. Int. Urol. Nephrol. **38**, 79–85 (2006)
9. Danciu, I., Cowan, J.D., Basford, M., Wang, X., Saip, A., Osgood, S., Shirey-Rice, J., Kirby, J., Harris, P.A.: Secondary use of clinical data: the Vanderbilt approach. J. Biomed. Inform. **52**, 28–35 (2014)
10. Xu, Z., Burke, R.P., Lee, C.P., Baucom, R.B., Poulose, B.K., Abramson, R.G., Landman, B.A.: Efficient abdominal segmentation on clinically acquired CT with SIMPLE context learning. Proc. SPIE Int. Soc. Opt. Eng. **9413**, 94130L (2015)
11. McAuliffe, M.J., Lalonde, F.M., McGarry, D., Gandler, W., Csaky, K., Trus, B.L.: Medical image processing, analysis and visualization in clinical research. In: 14th IEEE Symposium on Computer-Based Medical Systems (CBMS 2001), Proceedings, pp. 381–386. IEEE (2001)
12. Criminisi, A., Jamie, S., Konukoglu, E.: Decision forests: a unified framework for classification, regression, density estimation, manifold learning and semi-supervised learning. Found. Trends® Comput. Graph Vis. **7.2**(3), 81–227 (2012)
13. Modat, M., Ridgway, G.R., Taylor, Z.A., Lehmann, M., Barnes, J., Hawkes, D.J., Fox, N.C., Ourselin, S.: Fast free-form deformation using graphics processing units. Comput. Methods Programs Biomed. **98**, 278–284 (2010)
14. Burke, R.P., Xu, Z., Lee, C.P., Baucom, R.B., Poulose, B.K., Abramson, R.G., Landman, B.A.: Multi-atlas segmentation for abdominal organs with gaussian mixture models. Proc. SPIE Int. Soc. Opt. Eng. **9417**, 941707 (2015)

15. Wang, H., Suh, J.W., Das, S.R., Pluta, J.B., Craige, C., Yushkevich, P.A.: Multi-atlas segmentation with joint label fusion. IEEE Trans. Pattern Anal. Mach. Intell. **35**, 611–623 (2013)

16. Kerschnitzki, M., Kollmannsberger, P., Burghammer, M., Duda, G.N., Weinkamer, R., Wagermaier, W., Fratzl, P.: Architecture of the osteocyte network correlates with bone material quality. J. Bone Miner. Res. **28**, 1837–1845 (2013)

17. Elbahnasy, A.M., Shalhav, A.L., Hoenig, D.M., Elashry, O.M., Smith, D.S., McDougall, E.M., Clayman, R.V.: Lower caliceal stone clearance after shock wave lithotripsy or ureteroscopy: the impact of lower pole radiographic anatomy. J. Urol. **159**, 676–682 (1998)

18. Chew, B.H., Brotherhood, H.L., Sur, R.L., Wang, A.Q., Knudsen, B.E., Yong, C., Marien, T., Miller, N.L., Krambeck, A.E., Charchenko, C., Humphreys, M.R.: Natural history, complications and re-intervention rates of asymptomatic residual stone fragments after ureteroscopy: a report from the EDGE research consortium. J. Urol. **195**, 982–986 (2016)

19. Liu, J., Wang, S., Turkbey, E.B., Linguraru, M.G., Yao, J., Summers, R.M.: Computer-aided detection of renal calculi from noncontrast CT images using TV-flow and MSER features. Med. Phys. **42**, 144–153 (2015)

20. Liu, J., Wang, S., Linguraru, M.G., Yao, J., Summers, R.M.: Computer-aided detection of exophytic renal lesions on non-contrast CT images. Med. Image Anal. **19**, 15–29 (2015)

21. Will, S., Martirosian, P., Wurslin, C., Schick, F.: Automated segmentation and volumetric analysis of renal cortex, medulla, and pelvis based on non-contrast-enhanced T1- and T2-weighted MR images. MAGMA **27**, 445–454 (2014)

Local Phase-Based Learning for Needle Detection and Localization in 3D Ultrasound

Cosmas Mwikirize[1]($\boxtimes$), John L. Nosher[2], and Ilker Hacihaliloglu[1,2]

[1] Department of Biomedical Engineering, Rutgers University, Piscataway, USA
cosmas.mwikirize@rutgers.edu
[2] Department of Radiology, Rutgers Robert Wood Johnson Medical School,
New Brunswick, USA

Abstract. Described here is a novel method for automatic detection and enhancement of needles under 3D ultrasound guidance. We develop a detector consisting of a linear learning-based pixel classifier that utilizes Histogram of Oriented Gradients descriptors extracted from local phase projections. The detector automatically identifies slices of the volume that contain needle data, reducing the needle search space. Needle tip enhancement is performed on a projection of the extracted sub-volume, followed by automatic tip localization using spatially distributed image statistics within the trajectory constrained region. Evaluation of the proposed method on 40 volumes of *ex vivo* bovine tissue shows 88% detection precision, 98% recall rate, mean classification time per slice of 0.06 s and mean tip localization error of 0.44 ± 0.13 mm. The promising results indicate potential of the method for further evaluation on clinical pain management procedures.

1 Introduction

Ultrasound (US) guidance for regional anesthesia has gained popularity in clinical practice because of its radiation-free, low-cost and real-time nature. With two-dimensional (2D) US, which is the current standard, it is often difficult to align the needle with the scan plane. Needle localization is even more difficult for deep or steep insertions. This may impair therapeutic efficacy or cause injury. To address this challenge, three-dimensional (3D) US has emerged as a viable alternative [1]. 3D US permits simultaneous multi-planar visualization of the needle without probe adjustment, hence orientation of the needle with respect to the scan plane need not be perfect. However, needle visibility in 3D US is affected by low dimension of the needle with respect to the US volume, signal attenuation, high intensity artifacts and speckle noise.

Previously, algorithms for needle enhancement and localization in 3D US were reported. These include: the 3D Hough transform (HT) [2], projection-based methods such as parallel integration projection (PIP) [3] and iterative model-fitting methods based on the random sample consensus (RANSAC) algorithm [4]. These methods generally suffer from computational complexity due to the large amount of volume data that must be processed [5]. Further, since these methods

© Springer International Publishing AG 2017
M.J. Cardoso et al. (Eds.): CARE/CLIP 2017, LNCS 10550, pp. 108–115, 2017.
DOI: 10.1007/978-3-319-67543-5_10

are intensity-based, challenges may arise under difficult imaging conditions or in the presence of high intensity US imaging artifacts.

Although the RANSAC based ROI-RK method proposed in [4,5] reduces calculation time, it is not robust to high intensity artifacts and steep insertion angles. The limitations of intensity-based methods can be overcome with the use of local phase features. A qualitative comparison of local phase, HT and RANSAC based needle-axis localization is presented in Fig. 1, where we observe that when the only high intensity feature present is the needle, all methods give accurate localization, short of which only local phase features consistently yield accurate localization. In [6], oscillation of a needle stylet was modeled into a projection-based localization framework, providing a more robust solution. However, oscillating the stylet during US guided needle insertion is difficult in a single operator scenario, especially for shallow angles.

Recently, a robust, intensity-invariant algorithm for needle enhancement and localization in 2D US was proposed [7]. Needle shaft and tip were enhanced by incorporating US signal transmission models in an optimization problem. The needle trajectory was estimated from local phase-based projections of the enhanced B-mode image [8]. However, incorrect tip localization arose when high intensity soft tissue artifacts were present along the needle trajectory. The algorithm also required proper alignment of the needle with the scan plane. In this paper, we address the limitations in [7] by extending this promising method

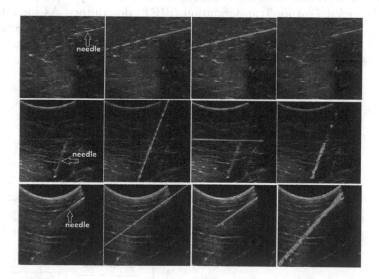

Fig. 1. Comparison of local phase, Hough transform and RANSAC based needle-axis localization. First column: 2D B-mode image. Second column-fourth column: Needle-axis localization (green) from local-phase, Hough transform and RANSAC respectively. When the needle is wholly conspicuous (top row), all methods give correct needle trajectory. When the needle shaft is broken or high intensity artifacts are present in the image, only the local phase-based method consistently gives accurate results. (Color figure online)

to 3D. Our main contributions are: (1) A learning based classifier that utilizes local phase descriptors to detect needle-containing slices in the US volume. (2) A technique that computes multi-planar reconstructions for needle tip localization in 3D. Our specific clinical focus is needle guidance in spinal injections such as lumbar facet joint and medial branch blocks in obese patients. Preliminary qualitative and quantitative validation results on *ex vivo* volumes demonstrate that our method is robust and has a low execution time, making it suitable for clinical evaluation in these pain management procedures.

2   Methods

We propose a two-stage framework illustrated in Fig. 2. We first detect slices (2D frames acquired from a motorized 3D transducer) with needle data. This is followed by needle enhancement and multi-planar tip localization. The following sub-sections describe this process in detail.

2.1   Needle Detection

Previously, locally normalized histograms of oriented gradients (HOG) descriptors were shown to be efficient at capturing gradient information [9]. They are also invariant to translations or rotations, demonstrating performance similar to Scale Invariant Feature Transformation (SIFT) descriptors. As such, locally normalized HOG descriptors make robust feature sets for needle detection. In our design, we extract intensity-invariant local phase descriptors and use them to derive HOG descriptors.

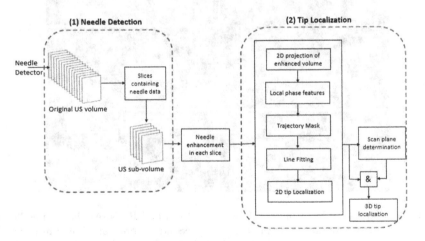

Fig. 2. Block diagram of the proposed approach. (1) A needle detector is used to classify slices that contain needle data, which are then compiled into a sub-volume as described in Sect. 2.1. (2) Needle tip localization is performed on the sub-volume after enhancement of needle data. The enhancement and localization processes are described in Sects. 2.2 and 2.3 respectively.

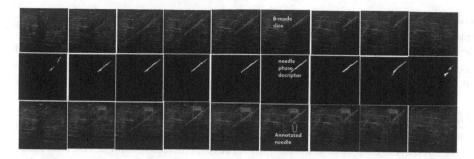

Fig. 3. The needle detection process. Top-row: B-mode US slices constituent of US_{volume}. The original volume comprised of 41 slices. Here, we show only 7 slices containing needle data, sandwiched between two slices (first and last columns) without needle data. Middle row: Respective $NPD(x,y)$ images. The slices with needle data possess a salient straight feature with minimum bending. The slices without needle data lack such features. Bottom row: Slice classification results after running the detector. The classification accuracy here was 100%.

Local Phase Descriptors for Needles: We apply orientation tuned intensity-invariant local phase filter banks to each slice of the 3D volume (hereafter denoted as US_{volume}) to extract a needle phase descriptor, hereafter denoted as $NPD(x,y)$. The filter banks are constructed from 2D Log-Gabor filters, whose parameters are selected automatically using the framework proposed in [8]. It is assumed that the insertion side of the needle is known *a priori*, and the calculation is limited to an automatically selected region of interest (ROI) on the insertion side. It is expected that the ROI contains a visible part of the shaft. The output of the filter operation gives a phase-based descriptor called phase symmetry, $PS(x,y)$, which is used as an input to the Maximum Likelihood Estimation SAmple Consensus algorithm (MLESAC) [10]. We use MLESAC to prune false positive pixels and connect inliers to yield $NPD(x,y)$. Figure 3 shows examples of slices with and without $NPD(x,y)$. Investigating Fig. 3 (first and last columns), we note that slices without needle data do not contain $NPD(x,y)$, while slices with needle data (middle 7 columns) possess $NPD(x,y)$, existing as bright intensity straight features, commensurate with a rigid needle.

Detector Architecture: For details of the HOG algorithm, we refer the reader to [9]. Specifically, we use L_2-Hys (Lowe-style clipped L_2-norm) contrast normalization on overlapping 3×3 cell blocks of 4×4 pixel cells: From the unnormalized descriptor vector $\mathbf{v}$, L_2-Hys is determined by clipping the L_2-norm, $\mathbf{v} \to \mathbf{v}/\sqrt{\| \mathbf{v} \|_2^2 + \epsilon^2}$ where ϵ is a small constant. This normalization is done to achieve invariance to geometric transformations. HOG computation is performed using a 64×128 sliding detection window, and the resulting descriptor is fed to a linear support vector machine (SVM) baseline classifier.

The detector is applied to each of the slices in US_{volume} after preprocessing to elicit needle phase descriptors similar to those used in training the detector. The resulting sub-volume, US^*_{volume}, consists of only slices that contain needle data.

Volume reduction saves computing load in the needle enhancement and localization steps that follow. It also removes slices that have artifacts which would degrade needle enhancement. Figure 3 (bottom row) illustrates an example of needle detection from volume data. Detected needles are shown with rectangular annotation.

2.2   Needle Enhancement

The goal of this step is to remove speckle, reverse attenuation effects, and minimize the effect of artifacts in the sub-volume US^*_{volume} so as to improve visibility of the needle shaft and tip. We design our approach to suit tip localization for in-plane insertion. In [7], it was shown that the needle tip and shaft can be enhanced by modeling US signal transmission using L_1-norm based contextual regularization. We follow a similar approach, where US signal transmission in each slice is modeled as $S(x, y) = S_t(x, y)S_e(x, y) + (1 - S_t(x, y))\kappa$. Here, $S(x, y)$ is a slice in US^*_{volume}, $S_t(x, y)$ is the signal transmission map, $S_e(x, y)$ is the desired enhanced image while κ is the average intensity of the tissue surrounding the needle in attenuated regions. $S_t(x, y)$ is obtained by minimizing the objective function:

$$\frac{\lambda}{2} \parallel S_t(x, y) - S_a(x, y) \parallel_2^2 + \sum_{i \in \zeta} \parallel \Gamma_i \circ (R_i \star S_t(x, y)) \parallel_1 \tag{1}$$

Here, $S_a(x, y)$ is a patch-wise transmission function representing boundary constraints imposed on the image by attenuation and orientation of the needle, ζ is an index set of image pixels, $\circ$ is element wise multiplication, and $\star$ is a convolution operator. R_i a bank of high order differential filters consisting of eight Kirsch filters and one Laplacian filter, and Γ_i is a weighting matrix calculated from $\Gamma_i(x, y) = exp(- \mid R_i(x, y) \star S(x, y) \mid^2)$. Details of how $S_a(x, y)$ is obtained are presented in [7]. After calculating $S_t(x, y)$ using (1), $S_e(x, y)$ is extracted from:

$$S_e(x, y) = [(S(x, y) - \kappa)/[max(S_t(x, y), \varepsilon)]^\rho] + \kappa \tag{2}$$

Here, ε is a small constant and ρ is related to the attenuation co-efficient of the tissue. To minimize the effect of high intensity artifacts aligned with the needle trajectory, each enhanced slice is subjected to a Top-hat filter operation using a linear structuring element. The final enhanced slices constitute the enhanced sub-volume denoted as USE^*_{volume}.

2.3   Tip Localization

In our workflow, the needle tip location is displayed in two planar visualizations, parallel and normal to the needle insertion direction. We consider a 3D US volume where x, y, z denote the lateral, axial and elevation directions respectively (Fig. 4). Our interest is determining $\Omega(x', y', z', \chi)$, the 3D tip location, where χ is the characteristic intensity of the tip in USE^*_{volume}.

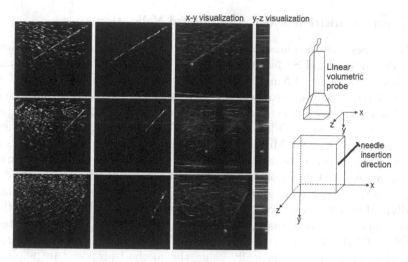

Fig. 4. The tip localization process. First column: $P_{x,y}$ image. Second column: $PE(x,y)$ image. The automatically localized tip (red) is overlaid on x–y (third column) and y–z (fourth column) slices, which jointly give tip location in 3D. The green cross represents the expert localized tip. Fifth column: 3D imaging coordinates. Top row: moderate insertion angle and needle aligned with US beam. Middle row: moderate insertion angle and needle not aligned with US beam. Bottom row: steep insertion angle and needle aligned with US beam. (Color figure online)

2D Tip Localization: If needle insertion is in the y–z plane, then the x–y plane is parallel to the needle insertion direction. We determine x' and y' from a projection $P_{x,y}$ since x' and y' have the same value in all slices. $P_{x,y}$ is calculated as the maximum intensity projection (MIP) of USE^{*}_{volume}, by extracting maximum intensity values along optical paths in the z direction. From this projection, the needle tip is localized following the algorithm in [8]. In summary, we determine the phase symmetry $PS(x,y)$ of $P_{x,y}$ in a region limited to the needle trajectory, apply the MLESAC algorithm for inlier detection and geometrical optimization, followed by feature extraction on the resultant point cloud using a combination of spatially distributed image statistics which enhance the needle tip. This yields the projection enhanced needle image denoted as $PE(x,y)$. (x',y') is determined from the first maximum intensity pixel at the distal end of the needle trajectory in $PE(x,y)$.

Scan Plane Determination: In this context, scan plane means the slice containing the needle tip, which is the most advanced portion of the needle in the elevation (z) direction of the volume. The scan plane is determined by calculating $\sum_{i=-\gamma}^{+\gamma} \sum_{j=-\gamma}^{+\gamma} I(x'+i, y'+j)$, the sum of pixel intensities in a bounded square patch of length 2γ centered at (x',y') in each slice within USE^{*}_{volume}. The scan plane is estimated as the slice with the maximum intensity sum. The result gives us z'. Figure 4 shows the tip localization process and qualitative results for different imaging conditions as well as the imaging coordinates used during tip localization.

2.4   Data Acquisition and Experimental Validation

3D US volumes were acquired using the SonixTouch system (Analogic Corporation, Peabody, MA, USA) equipped with a 4DL14-5/38 broadband volumetric probe. A 17-gauge (1.5 mm diameter, 90 mm length) Tuohy epidural needle (Arrow International, Reading, PA, USA) was inserted into freshly excised bovine tissue. The transducer motor was automatically controlled during insertion to achieve a Field of View (FOV) of 10° for sweeps of 0.244° per frame and 41 frames per volume. Multiple experiments were performed at various needle depths (40–80 mm) and orientations (30°–70°) with the needle in a native axial/elevation (y–z) direction of the volume. A total of 80 volumes were collected. The US system settings were fixed for all imaging sessions. The volumes were divided into 2 sets without overlap: 40 for training and 40 for validation.

The proposed method was implemented in MATLAB on a 3.6 GHz Intel(R) Core™ i7 CPU, 16 GB RAM Windows PC. The Log-Gabor filter parameters were determined automatically using the method proposed in [8]. In (2), $\kappa = 0.5 \times I_{max}$, where I_{max} is the maximum intensity in $S(x,y)$, $\rho = 2$ and $\varepsilon = 0.0005$. These values were empirically determined and fixed during validation. For the training dataset, 150 positive and 100 negative samples for $NPD(x,y)$ were manually selected. Performance of the needle detector was evaluated by calculating Precision (P) and Recall Rate (RR), where $P = True\ Positive/(True\ Positive + False\ Positive)$ and $RR = True\ Positive/(True\ Positive + False\ Negative)$. To determine localization accuracy, the ground truth tip location was segmented manually by an expert user in volumes where the tip was visible. Tip localization error was determined by calculating the Euclidean Distance (ED) between the automatically localized tip and the manually segmented tip.

3   Results

Qualitative results (Fig. 4) show that our method gives accurate tip localization for moderate to steep insertion angles, including cases when the shaft is discontinuous (Fig. 4 middle and bottom rows). Quantitative results revealed average precision of 88%, recall rate of 98%, detector execution time (per slice) of 0.06 s, overall execution time (for both slice detection and tip localization) of 3.5 s, tip localization error of 0.44 ± 0.13 mm and maximum localization error of 1.62 mm.

4   Discussion and Conclusions

We have proposed a novel learning-based method for automatic detection and localization of needles in US volumes. The low slice classification time potentially suits real-time applications and can complement previous approaches such as those reported in [2–6]. Considering the anatomy of our focus application (medial branch nerves are typically about 1 mm in diameter), a tip localization error of less than 1 mm is clinically acceptable. In [7], analysis of US data from porcine, bovine, kidney and liver tissue showed that local phase features are not affected by the intensity variations caused by different tissue types. Since the detector uses HOG descriptors derived from local phase features, detection accuracy is independent of tissue type. On account of including needle data from pertinent slices, accurate tip localization is possible when the needle is misaligned with the scan plane. The sufficiently high recall rate demonstrates that the detected volume always contains sufficient needle data to support the localization process.

The method is validated on epidural needles with minimal bending. For enhancement of bending needles, the proposed model can be updated by incorporating bending information into the framework. In future, we will investigate automating parameter selection for the algorithm, performance of the proposed method on needles of different gauges, real-time implementation of the proposed method, and a 3D classifier, in which needle detection is performed in a single extraction step applied to the entire volume.

References

1. Clendenen, S.R., Riutort, K., Ladlie, B.L., Robards, C., Franco, C.D., Greengrass, R.A.: Real-time three-dimensional ultrasound-assisted axillary plexus block defines soft tissue planes. Anesth. Analg. **108**, 1347–50 (2009)
2. Zhou, H., Qiu, W., Ding, M., Zhang, S.: Automatic needle segmentation in 3D ultrasound images using 3D improved Hough transform. In: Proceedings of SPIE Medical Imaging, vol. 6918, pp. 691821-1–691821-9 (2008)
3. Barva, M., Uhercik, M., Mari, J.M., Kybic, J., Duhamel, J.R., Liebgott, H., Hlavac, V., Cachard, C.: Parallel integral projection transform for straight electrode localization in 3-D ultrasound images. IEEE Trans. Ultrason. Ferroelectr. Freq. Control **55**(7), 1559–1569 (2008)
4. Zhao, Y., Bernard, A., Cachard, C., Liebgott, H.: Biopsy needle localization and tracking using ROI-RK method. Abstr. Appl. Anal. **2014**, 1–7 (2014). Article ID 973147. doi:10.1155/2014/973147
5. Zhao, Y., Shen, Y., Bernard, A., Cachard, C., Liebgott, H.: Evaluation and comparison of current biopsy needle localization and tracking methods using 3D ultrasound. Ultrasonics **73**, 206–20 (2017)
6. Beigi, P., Rohling, R., Salcudean, T., Lessoway, V.A., Ng, G.C.: Needle trajectory and tip localization in real-time 3-D ultrasound using a moving stylus. Ultrasound Med. Biol. **41**(7), 2057–2070 (2015)
7. Mwikirize, C., Nosher, J.L., Hacihaliloglu, I.: Enhancement of needle tip and shaft from 2D ultrasound using signal transmission maps. In: Ourselin, S., Joskowicz, L., Sabuncu, M.R., Unal, G., Wells, W. (eds.) MICCAI 2016. LNCS, vol. 9900, pp. 362–369. Springer, Cham (2016). doi:10.1007/978-3-319-46720-7_42
8. Hacihaliloglu, I., Beigi, P., Ng, G., Rohling, R.N., Salcudean, S., Abolmaesumi, P.: Projection-based phase features for localization of a needle tip in 2D curvilinear ultrasound. In: Navab, N., Hornegger, J., Wells, W.M., Frangi, A.F. (eds.) MICCAI 2015. LNCS, vol. 9349, pp. 347–354. Springer, Cham (2015). doi:10.1007/978-3-319-24553-9_43
9. Dalal, N., Triggs, B.: Histograms of oriented gradients for human detection. In: IEEE CVPR (2005)
10. Torr, P.H.S., Zisserman, A.: MLESAC: a new robust estimator with application to estimating image geometry. Comput. Vis. Image Underst. **78**(1), 138–156 (2000)

Intracranial Volume Quantification from 3D Photography

Liyun Tu[1(✉)], Antonio R. Porras[1], Scott Ensel[1], Deki Tsering[2], Beatriz Paniagua[3],
Andinet Enquobahrie[3], Albert Oh[4], Robert Keating[2], Gary F. Rogers[4],
and Marius George Linguraru[1,5]

[1] Sheikh Zayed Institute for Pediatric Surgical Innovation,
Children's National Health System, Washington DC, USA
tuliyun@gmail.com

[2] Division of Neurosurgery, Children's National Health System, Washington DC, USA

[3] Kitware Inc., Carrboro, NC, USA

[4] Division of Plastic and Reconstructive Surgery, Children's National Health System,
Washington DC, USA

[5] School of Medicine and Health Sciences, George Washington University,
Washington DC, USA

Abstract. 3D photography offers non-invasive, radiation-free, and anesthetic-free evaluation of craniofacial morphology. However, intracranial volume (ICV) quantification is not possible with current non-invasive imaging systems in order to evaluate brain development in children with cranial pathology. The aim of this study is to develop an automated, radiation-free framework to estimate ICV. Pairs of computed tomography (CT) images and 3D photographs were aligned using registration. We used the real ICV calculated from the CTs and the head volumes from their corresponding 3D photographs to create a regression model. Then, a template 3D photograph was selected as a reference from the data, and a set of landmarks defining the cranial vault were detected automatically on that template. Given the 3D photograph of a new patient, it was registered to the template to estimate the cranial vault area. After obtaining the head volume, the regression model was then used to estimate the ICV. Experiments showed that our volume regression model predicted ICV from head volumes with an average error of 5.81 ± 3.07% and a correlation (R^2) of 0.96. We also demonstrated that our automated framework quantified ICV from 3D photography with an average error of 7.02 ± 7.76%, a correlation (R^2) of 0.94, and an average estimation error for the position of the cranial base landmarks of 11.39 ± 4.3 mm.

Keywords: 3D photography · Computed tomography · Intracranial volume quantification · Registration

1 Introduction

Cranial volume analysis is important to assess craniofacial development and pathology. Specifically, intracranial volume (ICV) plays an essential role in the assessment of craniosynostosis and the decision factors for treatment, since the early fusion of the

M.J. Cardoso et al. (Eds.): CARE/CLIP 2017, LNCS 10550, pp. 116–123, 2017.
DOI: 10.1007/978-3-319-67543-5_11

cranial sutures can alter brain growth [1, 2]. In addition, longitudinal assessment of ICV is equally important after surgical treatment to evaluate the outcome of the intervention.

Most methods to quantify ICV are based on brain segmentation from computed tomography (CT) [3] or magnetic resonance imaging (MRI) scans [4]. However, CT involves radiation and MRI typically requires sedation or anesthesia for young children. Due to concerns about the risks of radiation and/or sedation in these patients, 3D photography has become an increasingly attractive modality to assess head volume, since it offers radiation-free, non-invasive, and anesthetic-free imaging [5, 6].

Wilbrand et al. [7] demonstrated that 3D photography has great potential to track and quantify the clinical course of surgical correction of craniosynostosis. Meulstee et al. [8] used 3D photography to evaluate the cranial shape to identify craniosynostosis. Freudl-sperger et al. [9] used 3D photography to capture pre- and post-operative scans of children with metopic craniosynostosis to compare head volume (HV) changes before and after surgery. However, these works focus on the head volume and shape, which do not measure the ICV (volume inside the cranial vault).

The aim of this study is to automatically quantify the ICV from 3D photography. First, we register a set of paired CT images and 3D photographs from the same patients to create a regression model that estimates the ICV (obtained from CT) from the HV measured from the 3D photography. We then use the regression model in conjunction with the 3D photograph of a new patient, for which we automatically measure the HV using registration to a 3D photograph reference template. The resulting framework allows us to automatically quantify the ICV from 3D photography to monitor patients with cranial pathology.

2   Materials and Methods

In the following sections, we will describe each component of our framework to fully automatic estimate ICV from 3D photography (see Fig. 1).

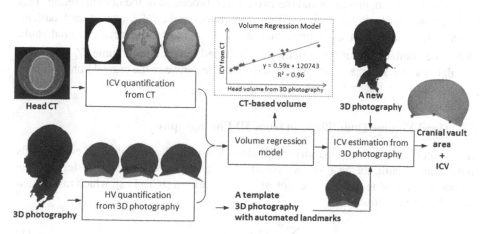

Fig. 1. Schematic of the proposed framework. ICV: intracranial volume. HV: head volume. The methods used for each of the boxes in this figure are detailed in Sect. 2 of the paper.

2.1 Data Description

Pairs of retrospective head CT imaging and 3D photography were collected by our institution from 14 subjects (average age 47 ± 66 months, range 2–199 months) with a variety of craniofacial pathologies (e.g., craniosynostosis and velopharyngeal insufficiency). All 3D photographs were taken at an average of 13 ± 18 days (range 0–49 days) from their corresponding CTs. CT image in-plane resolution ranged 0.26–0.49 mm, with axial spacing smaller or equal to 5 mm. 3D photographs were acquired using the 3dMDhead System (3dMD, Atlanta, GA). In the next sections, we will refer to this dataset as Φ_{pairs}.

In addition, we also collected an independent dataset $\Phi_{singles}$ of 3D photographs from 14 new patients (average age 88 ± 62 months, range 7–193 months) with craniofacial pathologies without paired CT.

2.2 Intracranial Volume Quantification from CT

To register a 3D photograph to its paired CT image (Φ_{pairs} dataset), we first created a 3D surface representing the patient's head (including the skin) from CT. We segmented the image areas with signal intensity higher than −200 Hounsfield units (HU), which separates the whole head from the background. We used morphological opening to isolate the inner tissues and we extracted the largest connected component, which provided a binary mask defining the patient's head. The marching cubes algorithm [10] was used to reconstruct the head surface from the image, which resulted in a single layered triangular mesh of the head.

The cranial bones were extracted from CT using the approach described in [3, 11]. In summary, a binary image with the bone structures was obtained from CT by thresholding at HU > 100. This binary image was then registered (optimizing translation, rotation and scaling) to a reference template in which a set of 4 landmarks were manually placed at the nasion, opisthion and the two clinoid processes of the dorsum sellae. This registration identified the location of these landmarks in the CT image of each patient, which define the two planes at the cranial base that we used to extract the cranial vault. Given the cranial vault of the patient, the CT-based intracranial volume (V_{CT_ICV}) was calculated as the volume within the cranial vault (i.e. between the cranial bones and the planes defined by the cranial base landmarks).

2.3 Head Volume Quantification from 3D Photography

To extract the part of the head surface obtained from 3D photography that corresponds to the cranial vault, the head surface obtained from its paired CT was registered to the 3D photograph using the iterative closest point algorithm (ICP) [12], which minimized the following equation:

$$E = \sum_{i=0}^{N} |Tp_i - q_i|^2, \tag{1}$$

where p_i are the homogeneous coordinates of point i in the head surface extracted from CT, q_i are corresponding coordinates in the 3D photograph, N is the number of points on the surface from CT, and T is the rigid transformation estimated. Point correspondences were established by searching each point on the CT surface to locate its closest point in the 3D photograph.

After registration, the cranial base landmarks identified in the CT image were propagated to the 3D photograph using T. The head volume (V_{3D_HV}) from the 3D photograph was calculated as the volume between the head surface and the cranial base defined by the 4 cranial base landmarks, as illustrated in Fig. 2.

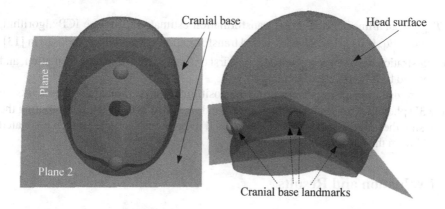

Fig. 2. Cranial vault area estimation for head volume measurement. The green surface represents the patient's head surface, which can be obtained from CT or 3D photograph. The cranial base (in purple) corresponds to two planes defined by the 4 cranial base landmarks at the nasion, opisthion and the two clinoid processes of the dorsum sellae. (Color figure online)

2.4   Intracranial Volume Estimation from 3D Photography

From the two volumes quantified in previous sections, V_{CT_ICV} and V_{3D_HV}, we built a linear regression model. This model will allow predicting the ICV given the HV calculated from the 3D photograph of a patient (V_{3D_HV}). In this section, we present a method to estimate V_{3D_HV} without the need of a paired CT image.

We selected a 3D photograph of a patient with a paired CT image as a reference template (R_{shape}) in which we located the cranial base landmarks ($R_{landmark}$) using its CT image as previously explained. Then, given the 3D photograph of a new patient (M_{shape}), we registered it to the reference template to estimate the location of the landmarks. Table 1 shows the proposed registration algorithm.

Table 1. Cranial base landmarks estimation via registration.

Input: R_{shape}, $R_{landmark}$, M_{shape}
Output: $M_{landmark}$
calculate an optimal affine transformation T_{affine}: $(R_{shape}) \mapsto M_{shape}$
transform the landmark $M'_{landmark} = T_{affine}$: $(R_{landmark})$
initialize the non-rigid transformation using $T_{affine}(R_{shape})$
calculate an optimal B-splines based transformation, T_{local}: $T_{affine}(R_{shape}) \mapsto M_{shape}$
estimate the landmark $M_{landmark} = T_{local}$: $(M'_{landmark})$

T_{affine} is an affine surface-based transformation estimated using the ICP algorithm, as shown in Eq. 1. T_{local} is a B-spline based transformation estimated as proposed in [13]. The registration between R_{shape} and M_{shape} is first optimized by affine transformation, and then refined by a non-rigid deformation.

This registration allows determining the position of the 4 cranial base landmarks on a new 3D photograph without using a corresponding CT image, and thus computing the HV. Using the volume regression model created in previous section, we then estimated the ICV from the calculated HV.

3   Evaluation and Results

The CT-based true intracranial volume (V_{CT_ICV}) and the head volume (V_{3D_HV}) from its corresponding 3D photograph in dataset Φ_{pairs} were computed to create a linear regression model as explained in Sect. 2.2. The model, which is shown in Fig. 3, yielded a clinically acceptable average volumetric error of $5.81 \pm 3.07\%$ and a correlation (R^2) of 0.96.

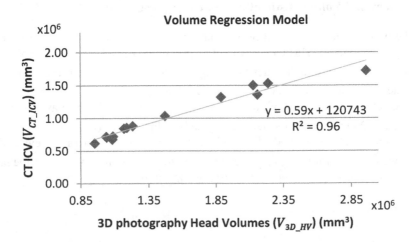

Fig. 3. Linear regression model predicting intracranial volume based on the automated head volume quantification from 3D photography.

We used the proposed framework to estimate the ICV (V_{3D_ICV}) using only the 3D photographs from the patients in Φ_{pairs}, and we compared the estimated values with the real ICV (V_{CT_ICV}) quantified from their paired CT images. We obtained an average volumetric error of $7.02 \pm 7.76\%$ and a correlation (R^2) of 0.94. In addition, we obtained an average estimation error for the position of the cranial base landmarks of 11.39 ± 4.3 mm. Figure 4 represents the Bland-Altman analysis [14] showing the agreement between V_{3D_ICV} and V_{CT_ICV}. There was one outlier that represents 31.67% of the error due to artifacts in the 3D photograph close to the neck area, which could be improved by a more efficient pre-processing. If we exclude this case the average volumetric error decreases to $5.16 \pm 3.63\%$. Next, we used a Wilcoxon rank-sum test to test whether the distribution of V_{3D_ICV} and V_{CT_ICV} were statistically different, obtaining a p-value of 0.91. Therefore, we could not reject the hypothesis that the ICV estimated from 3D photography has the same distribution than the true ICV estimated from CT imaging.

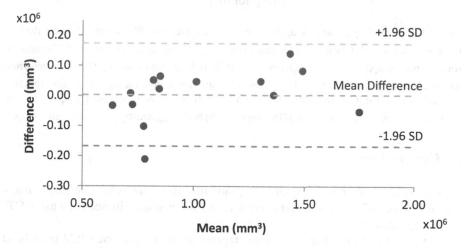

Fig. 4. Bland-Altman plot comparing the estimated ICV from 3D photography (V_{3D_ICV}) and the true ICV from CT (V_{CT_ICV}) for the patients in Φ_{pairs}.

Finally, we estimated the ICV from an independent dataset of 3D photographs ($\Phi_{singles}$) using the proposed framework. Figure 5 shows the ICV quantified from the 3D photographs of both datasets ($\Phi_{singles}$ and Φ_{pairs}) together with the true ICV from the CT images in Φ_{pairs}. We also calculated an age regression function of the form $y = \alpha x^\beta$ both for the true ICV volume from CT, and for the ICV estimated from 3D photography, where y is the ICV in mm^3 and x is the age of the patients in months. As it can be observed, the age regression functions are similar, indicating the potential to estimate ICV from 3D photography using our framework.

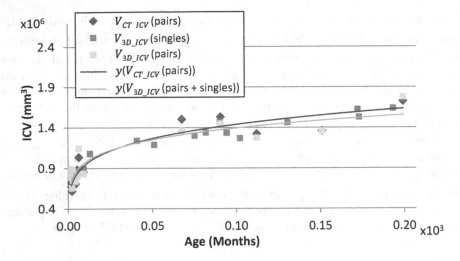

Fig. 5. Representation of the ICV against the age of the patients. Blue diamonds show the true ICV quantified from CT images for the cases from Φ_{pairs}. Green squares show the ICV estimated from 3D photography for the cases from Φ_{pairs}, while red squares show the ICV estimated from 3D photography for the cases in $\Phi_{singles}$. The blue line represents the age regression function estimated for the true ICV obtained from CT, while the magenta line represents the age regression function for the ICV estimated from 3D photography in both Φ_{pairs} and $\Phi_{singles}$. (Color figure online)

4   Conclusions

We proposed an automated, non-invasive, radiation-free framework to estimate intracranial volume (ICV) using 3D photography, and we evaluated its accuracy using CT-based measurements.

Experiments showed that our volume regression model predicted ICV from head volumes with an average error of $5.81 \pm 3.07\%$ and a correlation (R^2) of 0.96. We also demonstrated that our automated framework quantified ICV from 3D photography with an average error of $7.02 \pm 7.76\%$ (p-value = 0.91), a correlation (R^2) of 0.94, and an average estimation error for the position of the cranial base landmarks of 11.39 ± 4.3 mm.

Future work includes the validation of the proposed framework on a larger population. In addition, the framework can be extended to integrate cranial shape assessment, which will allow for a non-invasive longitudinal assessment of the surgical outcome for several craniofacial interventions.

Acknowledgements. This work was partly funded by the National Institutes of Health, Eunice Kennedy Shriver National Institute of Child Health and Human Development under grant NIH R42HD081712.

References

1. Anderson, P.J., Netherway, D.J., Abbott, A., David, D.J.: Intracranial volume measurement of metopic craniosynostosis. J. Craniofac. Surg. **15**(6), 1014–1016 (2004)
2. Paniagua, B., Emodi, O., Hill, J., Fishbaugh, J., Pimenta, L.A., Aylward, S.R., Andinet, E., Gerig, G., Gilmore, J., van Aalst, J.A., et al.: 3D of brain shape and volume after cranial vault remodeling surgery for craniosynostosis correction in infants. In: Proceeding of SPIE Medical Imaging, 2013, vol. 8672, p. 86720V (2013)
3. Mendoza, C.S., Safdar, N., Okada, K., Myers, E., Rogers, G.F., Linguraru, M.G.: Personalized assessment of craniosynostosis via statistical shape modeling. Med. Image Anal. **18**(4), 635–646 (2014)
4. Prastawa, M., Gilmore, J.H., Lin, W., Gerig, G.: Automatic segmentation of MR images of the developing newborn brain. Med. Image Anal. **9**(5), 457–466 (2005)
5. Ezaldein, H.H., Metzler, P., Persing, J.A., Steinbacher, D.M.: Three-dimensional orbital dysmorphology in metopic synostosis. J. Plast. Reconstr. Aesthetic Surg. **67**(7), 900–905 (2014)
6. Rodriguez-Florez, N., Göktekin, Ö.K., Bruse, J.L., Borghi, A., Angullia, F., Knoops, P.G., Tenhagen, M., O'Hara, J.L., Koudstaal, M.J., Schievano, S., et al.: Quantifying the effect of corrective surgery for trigonocephaly: a non-invasive, non-ionizing method using three-dimensional handheld scanning and statistical shape modeling. J. Cranio-Maxillofacial Surg. **45**(3), 387–394 (2017)
7. Wilbrand, J.-F., Szczukowski, A., Blecher, J.-C., Pons-Kuehnemann, J., Christophis, P., Howaldt, H.-P., Schaaf, H.: Objectification of cranial vault correction for craniosynostosis by three-dimensional photography. J. Cranio-Maxillofacial Surg. **40**(8), 726–730 (2012)
8. Meulstee, J.W., Verhamme, L.M., Borstlap, W.A., Van der Heijden, F., De Jong, G.A., Xi, T., Bergé, S.J., Delye, H., Maal, T.J.J.: A new method for three-dimensional evaluation of the cranial shape and the automatic identification of craniosynostosis using 3D stereophotogrammetry. Int. J. Oral Maxillofac. Surg. **46**(7), 819–826 (2017)
9. Freudlsperger, C., Steinmacher, S., Bächli, H., Somlo, E., Hoffmann, J., Engel, M.: Metopic synostosis: Measuring intracranial volume change following fronto-orbital advancement using three-dimensional photogrammetry. J. Cranio-Maxillofacial Surg. **43**(5), 593–598 (2015)
10. Lorensen, W.E., Cline, H.E.: Marching cubes: A high resolution 3D surface construction algorithm. Comput. Graph. (ACM) **21**(4), 163–169 (1987)
11. Porras, A.R., Zukic, D., Equobahrie, A., Rogers, G.F., Linguraru, M.G.: Personalized optimal planning for the surgical correction of metopic craniosynostosis. In: Shekhar, R., Wesarg, S., González Ballester, M.Á., Drechsler, K., Sato, Y., Erdt, M., Linguraru, M.G., Oyarzun Laura, C. (eds.) CLIP 2016. LNCS, vol. 9958, pp. 60–67. Springer, Cham (2016). doi: 10.1007/978-3-319-46472-5_8
12. Besl, P., McKay, N.: A method for registration of 3-D shapes. IEEE Trans. Pattern Anal. Mach. Intell. **14**(2), 239–256 (1992)
13. Rueckert, D., Sonoda, L.I., Hayes, C., Hill, D.L.G., Leach, M.O., Hawkes, D.J.: Nonrigid registration using free-form deformations: application to breast MR images. IEEE Trans. Med. Imaging **18**(8), 712–721 (1999)
14. Bland, J.M., Altman, D.: Statistical methods for assessing agreement between two methods of clinical measurement. Lancet **327**(8476), 307–310 (1986)

Automatic Near Real-Time Evaluation of 3D Ultrasound Scan Adequacy for Developmental Dysplasia of the Hip

Olivia Paserin[1(✉)], Kishore Mulpuri[2], Anthony Cooper[2], Antony J. Hodgson[3], and Rafeef Abugharbieh[1]

[1] Department of Electrical and Computer Engineering,
University of British Columbia, Vancouver, BC, Canada
opaserin@ece.ubc.ca
[2] Department of Orthopedic Surgery, British Columbia Children's Hospital,
Vancouver, BC, Canada
[3] Department of Mechanical Engineering, University of British Columbia,
Vancouver, BC, Canada

Abstract. Accurate detection and diagnosis of developmental dysplasia of the hip (DDH), a common hip instability condition among infants, relies heavily on acquiring adequate ultrasound (US) image data. Although 2D US is the standard modality used for DDH screening, 3D US has recently been considered as well. Presently there is no automatic method (or even a standardized manual method) capable of analyzing the US volume to determine whether that volume is adequate for extracting DDH metrics required for diagnosis. Scan adequacy in 2D has seen only one work on automation and there has been no work done on scan adequacy in 3D. We propose an automatic, near real-time method of assessing 3D ultrasound scans in developmental dysplasia screening and diagnostic applications using a convolutional neural network (CNN). Our classifier labels volumes as adequate or inadequate for subsequent interpretation based on the presence of hip anatomy needed for DDH diagnosis. We validate our approach on 40 datasets from 15 pediatric patients and demonstrate a classification rate of 100% with average processing time of just above 2 s per US volume. We expect automatic US scan adequacy assessment to have significant clinical impact with the potential to help in imaging standardization, improving efficiency of measuring DDH metrics, and improving accuracy of clinical decision making.

Keywords: 3D ultrasound · Developmental dysplasia of the hip · DDH · Convolutional neural networks · CNN · Scan adequacy · Real time

1 Introduction

Developmental dysplasia of the hip (DDH), a condition encompassing a spectrum of hip joint instabilities, is the most common hip disorder in infants. Due to its low cost, portability and absence of potentially harmful ionizing radiation,

© Springer International Publishing AG 2017
M.J. Cardoso et al. (Eds.): CARE/CLIP 2017, LNCS 10550, pp. 124–132, 2017.
DOI: 10.1007/978-3-319-67543-5_12

ultrasound (US) is the recommended imaging modality for DDH screening of the hip joint prior to ossification of the femoral head [1]. Although physical examination and US-based screening is routine in most countries, the standardization of these examinations remains a challenge. Typically, US images are manually acquired by an experienced radiologist or orthopedic surgeon as they search for key anatomical structures required to make certain measurements that lead to a diagnosis. Once judged to be adequate for interpretation, the US data are saved during the physical exam of the patient for later analysis when DDH metrics are extracted from the data (usually a manual process).

Accurate detection of hip joint instabilities and correct anatomical measurements needed for diagnosis heavily rely on the acquisition of high quality volumes that can successfully be used to complete the required tasks, namely extracting the α angle (the angle between the acetabular roof and the vertical cortex of the ilium), β angle (the angle between the labrum and the vertical cortex of the ilium), and femoral head coverage (the femoral head portion sitting in the acetabular cup of the hip joint) metrics for diagnosis. If no adequate data is collected during a patient visit, the patient must return for a subsequent appointment, resulting in both unnecessary effort, time and monetary costs. Obtaining adequate quality US acquisitions is a skill that becomes stronger with many years of clinical experience. For example, in Germany, special commissions control the quality of recorded US in an effort to reduce misdiagnoses [2]. However, when the quality of hip sonograms across 8 German states were tested in 2011, many hip sonography licenses were revoked because of their poor quality diagnoses using 2D US [3]. The reasons for misdiagnoses were: (1) US probe orientation errors; (2) incorrect anatomical interpretation; and (3) lack of adequacy check [2]. In 2011, refresher courses in Austria and Germany revealed the majority of mistakes made by 250 medical doctors who performing and classifying scans (64% of the tests) were due to wrong anatomical identification by the clinicians [2].

Correctly and efficiently guiding US to the desired anatomical locations and interpreting the images correctly are difficult tasks. A number of recent works addressed this issue in others fields, such as fetal abnormality screening [4,5] and cardiac imaging [6]. Only one group [7–9] has recently addressed 2D US scan adequacy for DDH. Quader [9] proposed a computational image analysis technique to automatically identify adequate images and subsequently extract dysplasia metrics in 2D. Although they produced excellent agreement with clinician adequacy classifications and reduced variability in the measured dysplasia metrics ($p < 0.05$), the computational time required for the 2D adequacy task was around 1 s per image [9]. This is not suitable for 3D volumes, as the time required for classification would add up to over 3 min of processing time per volume (205 slices total on our machine).

Computer-aided methods have shown good potential for improving detection rates of DDH from US. Very recently, quantification of infant hip using 3D US has shown promising results in improving diagnostic accuracy as the 3D scans capture the entire hip joint and are less prone to probe orientation errors compared to 2D scans [10]. Mabee [11] quantified 3D using the acetabular contact angle (ACA) and found it was significantly more reliable than 2D US α angle. Hareendranathan [12] proposed a semiautomatic algorithm to calculate ACA, and found that it reduced inter-observer and intra-observer variation in the calculation. Quader [13] also showed that a 3D alpha angle calculation may be significantly more reproducible than the conventional 2D measure. Subsequently, we focus on classifying 3D volumes although our implementation inherently solves the problem of 2D adequacy classification as well. To the best of our knowledge, no one has explored adequacy identification of US volumes used for making DDH measurements and our work is the first one to automate the volume standardization in DDH screening with 3D US.

2   Methods

We propose an automatic, near real-time technique for assessing 3D US scan adequacy for DDH in clinical settings using a trained convolutional neural network (CNN) to classify US volumes as adequate or inadequate for diagnostic interpretation. Our method performs slice by slice categorization of 2D images in search of the relevant anatomy of the hip needed for DDH metric extraction.

2.1   Materials and Experimental Setup

As part of our clinical study, we acquired 40 3D B-mode US volumes, made up of a total 8,200 slices, from 15 pediatric patients acquired by a team of two pediatric orthopedic surgeons at British Columbia Children's Hospital. We labelled a total of 3,078 slices from the dataset in order to maintain a balanced training set between adequate and inadequate samples, as there were 1,539 adequate slices within our 40 training volumes. The data was obtained as part of routine clinical care under appropriate institutional review board approval using a SonixTouch Q+ scanner (powered by Analogic) with a 4DL14-5/38 linear 4D transducer set at 7 MHz. Each acquired volume constituted 205 slices, with 6 slices per millimeter. All slices had a x-dimension of 38 mm and variable y-dimension of a minimum of 38 mm and were resized to 256×256 pixels to maintain consistency in the input dimensions to our neural network.

2.2   Ultrasound Scan Adequacy Criteria

We define an adequate 2D slice within a scan volume to be one containing the anatomical features necessary to extract the commonly used DDH metrics, namely the α angle, β angle, and femoral head coverage. Those anatomical features include the ilium, acetabulum, labrum, ischium and entire femoral head [9], as illustrated in Fig. 1. When a volume properly captures these features, the femoral head, a hypoechoic spherical structure, should be seen growing and shrinking in size across the encompassing slices with a region of interest spanning an average area of 8×8 mm, as 8 mm is the typical diameter of an infant's femoral head. Our adequacy criteria is rather straight forward: we hypothesize an adequate 3D scan to be one that contains sufficient number of adjacent adequate 2D frames. In our implementation, those were defined as spanning a minimum of 5 mm, corresponding to 30 slices on our machine. Additionally, we require inadequate slices to both precede and follow the adequate slices such that we are confident the entire hip joint is imaged without being cut off at the edge of the volume. In contrast, an inadequate scan volume will have a significantly lower number of adequate 2D slices (less than 30).

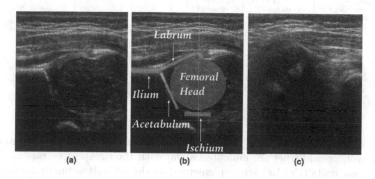

Fig. 1. 2D slice examples of (a) an adequate US slice, (b) the slice in (a) with the relevant anatomy needed for adequacy annotated on top, and (c) an inadequate US slice.

2.3   CNN Architecture

We implemented our network using Caffe [14] to classify 2D slices as adequate or inadequate based on the presence of the needed anatomy exemplified in Fig. 1. Classification based on 2D slices allows for training with fewer images due to significantly lower number of parameters needed for optimization during training compared to 3D CNN based classification. A block diagram of our network architecture is shown in Fig. 2.

The network receives a 227 × 227 image as input and begins with three convolutional layers. Each convolutional layer receives local receptive fields from the preceding layer and extracts a number of features depending on their number of filters. We employed rectified linear units (ReLUs) as activation functions between layers as they have been found to perform better than the traditional sigmoid function due to their sparse representations [15]. Max-pooling layers are used to nonlinearly downsample the resolution of the convolutional layers' feature maps. Inspired by the skipping layer implemented by Su [16], the outputs of both fully-connected layers are concatenated such that multi-scale features are preserved, since features in the second fully-connected layer (FC7) are more global that those in the first fully-connected layer (FC6). This concatenation avoids having the second fully-connected layer as a bottleneck for information propagation [16]. The final layer outputs the posterior probability for each class with a softmax loss function, which computes the multinomial logistic loss of

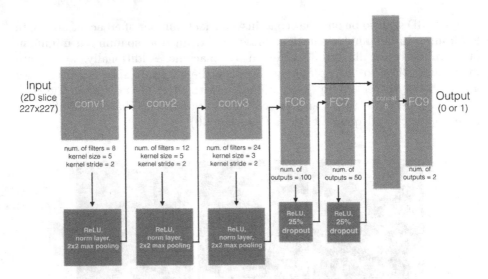

Fig. 2. Overview of the our CNN architecture. The number of filters, size, and stride of each convolutional kernel are indicated along with their respective rate of dropout. Rectified linear units (ReLUs) are implemented as the activation functions of all three convolutions along with normalization layers and 2×2 max-pooling. The convolutional layers are followed by two fully connected layers, each with a ReLU and 25% dropout, and then concatenated before the final softmax output layer.

the softmax of its inputs. This layer is conceptually the same as a softmax layer followed by a multinomial logistic loss layer, but provides a more numerically stable gradient.

2.4   Training

We split our dataset of 3,078 slices from 40 3D US volumes from 15 pediatric patients into a test set containing 20% of the subjects and used the remaining 80% for training. We performed 5-fold cross validation taking care to avoid mixing images from the same patient between training and validation groups. During training, we augmented each batch by cropping 227×227 sub-images, effectively reducing the field of view during training as a form of training data augmentation, as in [15]. We used a 25% dropout rate after both fully connected layers which we empirically found to be sufficient for avoiding overfit to the training set. We trained the net for 10 k iterations since both the test loss and test accuracy had stabilized by this time, and chose the net parameters with the lowest error on the validation set: namely momentums of 0.9 and 0.999, base learning rate of 0.001, and weight decay of 5e–8. *Adam*, a gradient-based optimization method similar to stochastic gradient descent proposed in [17], was used with gradients calculated by back-propagation and training was done on an 8-core Linux workstation with two Intel 3 GHz Xeon x5472 processors, an

Nvidia GeForce GTX 460 v2 GPU with 1 GB of GDDR5 VRAM, and 8 GB of host memory.

3   Results and Discussion

To assess the performance of our classifier, we tested on a validation dataset containing 20 unseen (by our network) US volumes from 5 new patients (10 adequate volumes, 10 inadequate volumes). For each test subject, we calculated and recorded the confidence for each class over all the slices in a volume. Our method implementation operates in near real-time, requiring only 9.9 ms for classifying one frame, adding up to only 2.03 s per volume (205 slices on our machine).

3.1   Criteria for Validation

It is important to note that there is no gold standard for clinical classification of US volumes, since 2D assessment is the clinical standard for DDH screening. To improve confidence in the adequacy labels of our test volumes, we used the only automatic 3D extraction method available [13] and ensured the relevant anatomy for both alpha angle (plane of the ilium and plane of the acetabulum) and femoral head coverage (plane of the ilium and femoral head) in 3D were successfully computed in all adequate volumes, as shown in Fig. 3. We found that

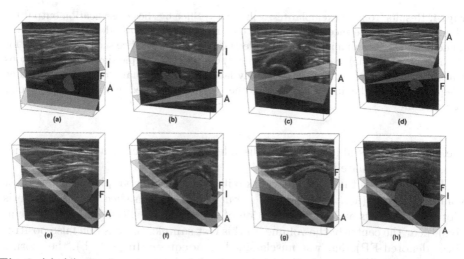

Fig. 3. (a)–(d) sample outputs resulting from running the automatic metric extraction of [13] on volumes classified as inadequate by our CNN. (e)–(h) sample outputs resulting from running the automatic metric extraction on volumes classified as adequate by our CNN. We found that the automatic algorithm was able to localize the relevant anatomy (femoral head in purple, plane of the ilium in blue, and plane of the acetabulum in green) in volumes classified as adequate by our CNN. (Color figure online)

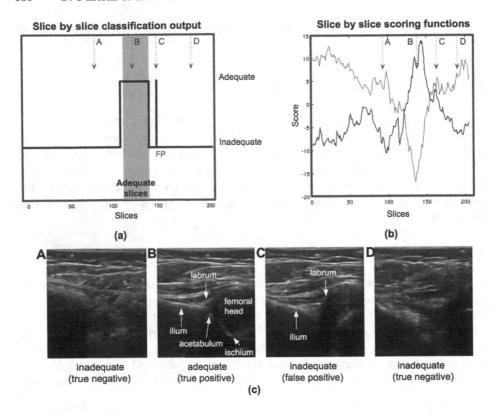

Fig. 4. Results from an exemplar test volume. (a) Slice by slice classification output (in blue). True adequate slices (in green) were correctly classified as adequate, while some inadequate slices were misclassified as adequate. (b) Slice by slice scoring functions for the adequate (in blue) and inadequate (in red) classes. (c) Sample slices at the locations marked in (b) (from left to right: correctly labeled as inadequate, correctly labeled as adequate, the misclassified slice, and another correctly labeled as inadequate). (Color figure online)

the algorithm was able to localize the relevant anatomical features in volumes classified as adequate by our CNN.

Figure 4 shows the sample network outputs from an example (adequate) test volume. In part (a), the classification output from each slice of the volume is plotted and shows a clear identification of the adequate slices (120 to 159 inclusive), near the centre of the volume. In this test sample, there is one false positive slice (denoted FP) that was misclassified as adequate. In part (b), the scoring functions for both adequate and inadequate class labels are plotted for the same test volume. The majority of slices show strong differences in scoring functions (expressing high confidence in the network's prediction) for the correct output class, with small differences occurring at the boundaries where inadequate slices become adequate slices and vice versa. The misclassified slice had a difference between scoring functions of less than one, indicating that the network was uncertain about the class for this image and chose an adequate label over an inadequate one with low confidence. This slice is shown in part (c), where it can be seen that the image has a visible ilium and labrum, but is missing the remaining acetabulum and ischium.

4 Conclusions

In this study, we proposed an CNN based automated method for classification of 3D US scan adequacy for application to DDH screening and diagnosis. Our network design allows for robust real-time inference crucial for real life clinical workflow. This promising approach may improve acquisitions, assist operators in volume interpretation, and allow the time-consuming step of extracting dysplasia metrics to be confidently deferred to off-line calculations resulting in better clinical management.

For our future work we will expand the size of our training set to include all 35 patients from our clinical study. We plan to investigate the differences in reliability and task time between novice and experienced sonographers/surgeons using our setup. Ultimately, we aim to design and test a fully automatic system that combines our proposed scan adequacy module with automatic DDH metric extraction.

References

1. Atweh, L., Kan, J.: Multimodality imaging of developmental dysplasia of the hip. Pediatr. Radiol. **43**(1), 166–171 (2013)
2. Graf, R., Mohajer, M., Florian, P.: Hip sonography update: quality-management, catastrophes - tips and tricks. Med. Ultrason. **15**(4), 299–303 (2013)
3. Tschauner, C., Matthissen, H.: Hip sonography with graf-method in newborns: checklists help to avoid mistakes. OUB J. **1**, 7–8 (2012)
4. Maraci, M., Bridge, C., Napolitano, R., Papageorghiou, A., Noble, A.: A framework for analysis of linear ultrasound videos to detect fetal presentation and heartbeat. Med. Image Anal. **37**, 22–36 (2017)
5. Rahmatullah, B., Papageorghiou, A., Noble, J.A.: Automated selection of standardized planes from ultrasound volume. In: Suzuki, K., Wang, F., Shen, D., Yan, P. (eds.) MLMI 2011. LNCS, vol. 7009, pp. 35–42. Springer, Heidelberg (2011). doi:10.1007/978-3-642-24319-6_5
6. Baumgartner, C.F., Kamnitsas, K., Matthew, J., Smith, S., Kainz, B., Rueckert, D.: Real-time standard scan plane detection and localisation in fetal ultrasound using fully convolutional neural networks. In: Ourselin, S., Joskowicz, L., Sabuncu, M.R., Unal, G., Wells, W. (eds.) MICCAI 2016. LNCS, vol. 9901, pp. 203–211. Springer, Cham (2016). doi:10.1007/978-3-319-46723-8_24
7. Quader, N., Hodgson, A., Mulpuri, K., Savage, T., Abugharbieh, A.: Automatic assessment of developmental dysplasia of the hip. In: IEEE 12th International Symposium on Biomedical Imaging (ISBI), pp. 13–16 (2015)
8. Quader, N., Schaeffer, E., Mulpuri, K., Cooper, A., Hodgson, A., Abugharbieh, R.: Automatic evaluation of scan adequacy and dysplasia metrics in 2D ultrasound images of the neonatal hip. Bone Joint J. **98–B**(sup. 21), 42 (2016)

9. Quader, N., Hodgson, A., Mulpuri, K., Schaeffer, E., Abugharbieh, R.: Automatic evaluation of scan adequacy and dysplasia metrics in 2-D ultrasound images of the neonatal hip. Ultras. Med. Biol. **43**(6), 1252–1262 (2017)
10. Jaremko, J., Mabee, M., Swami, V., Jamieson, L., Chow, K., Thompson, R.: Potential for change in US diagnosis of hip dysplasia solely caused by changes in probe orientation: patterns of alpha-angle variation revealed by using three-dimensional US. Radiology **273**(3), 870–878 (2014)
11. Mabee, M., Hareendranathan, A., Thompson, R., Dulai, S., Jaremko, J.: An index for diagnosing infant hip dysplasia using 3-D ultrasound: the acetabular contact angle. Pediatr. Radiol. **46**(7), 1023–1031 (2016)
12. Hareendranathan, A., Mabee, M., Punithakumar, K., Noga, M., Jaremko, J.: A technique for semiautomatic segmentation of echogenic structures in 3D ultrasound, applied to infant hip dysplasia. Int. J. Comput. Assist. Radiol. Surg. **11**(1), 31–42 (2015)
13. Quader, N., Hodgson, A., Mulpuri, K., Cooper, A., Abugharbieh, R.: Towards reliable automatic characterization of neonatal hip dysplasia from 3D ultrasound images. In: Ourselin, S., Joskowicz, L., Sabuncu, M.R., Unal, G., Wells, W. (eds.) MICCAI 2016. LNCS, vol. 9900, pp. 602–609. Springer, Cham (2016). doi:10.1007/978-3-319-46720-7_70
14. Jia, Y., Shelhamer, E., Donahue, J., Karayev, S., Long, J., Girshick, R., Guadarrama, S., Darrell, T.: Caffe: convolutional architecture for fast feature embedding. In: 22nd ACM International Conference on Multimedia, pp. 675–678 (2014)
15. Krizhevski, A., Sutskever, I., Hinton, G.: ImageNet classification with deep convolutional neural networks. In: Neural Information Processing Systems, pp. 1097–1105 (2012)
16. Su, Y., Wang, X., Tang, X.: Deep learning face representation from predicting 10,000 classes. In: Proceedings of the IEEE Conference on Computer Vision and Pattern Recognition, pp. 1891–1898 (2014)
17. Kingma, D., Ba, J.: Adam: A Method for Stochastic Optimization. Proceedings of the 3rd International Conference on Learning Representations. arXiv preprint arXiv:1412.6980 (2015)

Automatic Sentinel Lymph Node Localization in Head and Neck Cancer Using a Coupled Shape Model Algorithm

Florian Jung[1,2(✉)], Biebl-Rydlo Medea[1], Jean-François Daisne[3],
and Stefan Wesarg[1]

[1] Fraunhofer Institut Für Graphische Datenverarbeitung,
Fraunhoferstr. 5, 64283 Darmstadt, Germany
florian.jung@igd.fraunhofer.de
[2] GRIS, Technische Universität Darmstadt,
Fraunhoferstr. 5, 64283 Darmstadt, Germany
[3] Radiation Oncology Department, Université Catholique de Louvain,
CHU-UCL-Namur, Site Sainte-Elisabeth,
Place Louise Godin 15, 5000 Namur, Belgium

Abstract. The localization and analysis of the sentinel lymph node for patients diagnosed with cancer, has significant influence on the prognosis, outcome and treatment of the disease. We present a fully automatic approach to localize the sentinel lymph node and additional active nodes and determine their lymph node level on SPECT-CT data. This is a crucial prerequisite for the planning of radiation therapy or a surgical neck dissection. Our approach was evaluated on 17 lymph nodes. The detection rate of the lymph nodes was 94%; and 88% of the lymph nodes were correctly assigned to their corresponding lymph node level. The proposed algorithm targets a very important topic in clinical practice. The first results are already very promising. The next step has to be the evaluation on a larger data set.

Keywords: SPECT imaging · Sentinel lymph node detection · Lymph node level classification

1 Introduction

Every year, 600.000 new incidences of head and neck cancer are diagnosed with an annual patient death rate of 300.000 [11]. One of the most significant prognostic factors for the disease is the presence or absence of metastases in sentinel lymph nodes (SLN). Lymph nodes play a crucial role in the human immune system. In case a patient develops cancer, cancerous cells can be transported through the lymphatic system and finally infiltrate lymph nodes. From there the disease can further spread throughout the human body and infiltrate other lymph nodes or organs. These distant metastasis (m-staging) are within the most devastating prognosis for a patient. Any stage of the disease, even an early T1 or

© Springer International Publishing AG 2017
M.J. Cardoso et al. (Eds.): CARE/CLIP 2017, LNCS 10550, pp. 133–140, 2017.
DOI: 10.1007/978-3-319-67543-5_13

T2 staged cancer, is upstaged to stage 4, the worst possible classification, when a distant metastatis (M1) is diagnosed [8]. Therefore, the presence or absence of metastases within the SLN and other distant lymph nodes is one of the most significant prognostic factors in (Head and Neck) cancer.

In clinical practice different treatment approaches in head and neck cancer are followed, depending on the location and the stage of the disease. The most extreme forms of treatment are the *active waiting* and the *elective neck dissection* [12]. With the former approach repeated screenings of the patient are done, as long as it is not clear if a metastases has taken place. The idea is, to not expose the patient to a overtreatment. Later is the exact opposite. During an elective neck dissection all lymph nodes in the area around the metastatic lymph node are surgically removed. In many cases this leads to an overtreatment. On the other hand, studies have shown, that the overall survival rate is higher and the reoccurance rate of the tumor is lower [5]. In all cases, where not only the tumor, but the lymphatic system is treated as well, a localisation of the sentinel lymph node is crucial. In cases where a patient is treated with radiation therapy, a selective irradiation of the target volume of the lymph node area containing the SLN is practice by international clinical guidelines [3].

The detection of the sentinel lymph node can be achieved in different ways. One intervention uses blue dye, which is injected during surgery at the tumor site. The flow of the dye is observed and thereby the sentinel lymph node can be determined [4]. Another possible approach is the usage of SPECT-CT imaging to investigate a possible tumor spread. Currently, the common practice in clinical routine is to only visually inspect the SPECT-CT image data, the image data is not used for any further analysis.

In this paper we propose a novel method to fully automatically extract meta information about the patient's lymph nodes from the acquired SPECT and CT image data, which is useful for radiation therapy or a surgical neck dissection. After a short introduction of the methods of our approach (see Sect. 2), we describe the test setup and perform a quantitative evaluation on clinical data sets.

2   Methods

Our approach consists of three steps (although the CT-CT registration is optional). In the first step (Sect. 2.1) the lymph nodes are located within the CT image. The second step is an optional step (Sect. 2.2). If present, the SPECT-CT scan is registered to a planning CT scan with a higher resolution. The idea hereby is to use a higher resolution input for the third step. As the third step (Sect. 2.3), we use our coupled shape model algorithm (CoSMo [6]) to automatically detect the lymph node levels in the head and neck region. The lymph nodes located on the SPECT image data are then mapped to the lymph node levels determined by CoSMo. All of these steps are run without any user interaction and provide the clinician with the lymph node levels of all active nodes and can be used for further clinical procedures (Fig. 1).

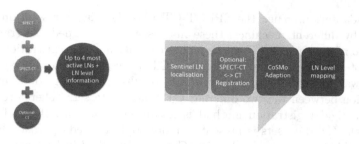

Fig. 1. The figure on the left side, shows which input is needed for the algorithm and what output it produces. The figure on the right visualizes the workflow of the lymph node localization process.

2.1 Lymph Node Localisation

Compared to CT image data, where the intensity values are already normalized by protocol, the SPECT image intensity values we observed were in range: [0, 65000]. After further observation it became clear, that no assumptions could be made about the intensity values of active lymph nodes, because there was a noticeable variance between different patients and different lymph nodes. Besides the obvious reason of different machines used for the acquisition of the scans, one of the reasons presumably is the fact that the intensity value of a lymph node depends on the uptake of the radioactive tracer and the time between the injection of the tracer and the image acquisition. But, not only the significant difference in intensity values yields a problem for an analysis, the huge amount of noise is an additional problem. As a result it can be considered that it is completely unfeasible to define a narrow intensity intervall beforehand wherein the lymph nodes reside.

We have designed a top-down approach to iteratively extract the active lymph nodes from the SPECT data. We generate a labelmap [7] of the SPECT image with a lower threshold t_i. Where $i \in [1, 10]$ and s_{max} is the maximum intensity value of the SPECT image data.

$$t_i = 10 * \sqrt{\frac{s_{max}}{i}} \qquad (1)$$

Within each iteration all labels are extracted from the label map. The 'hottest' structures always represents the tumor, while the others are considered as lymph nodes. It has been shown, that the monitoring of the 3 or 4 hottest nodes is sufficient for a correct staging [2]. So we are only interested in up to 4 active lymph nodes and for this reason we have added another termination condition, we automatically stop once we have found 4 active nodes,

2.2 Spect-CT - CT Registration

We added an additional optional step to the algorithm. In case a higher resolution planning CT is present (a radiation therapy planning CT), this can be used for

CoSMo adaptation. Since the SPECT-CT and the higher resolution CT are acquired by different machines, these images are not aligned. To transfer the information from the SPECT to the higher resolution CT a registration between the CT of the SPECT and the highres CT is required. The image data we received was taken using a fixation mask, resulting in a negligible amount of deformation between the two different CT image data sets. Therefore, for this scenario a rigid registration method is absolutely sufficient. If a deformation between the CT data sets is present, a more sophisticated approach has to be used. For this task an approach using CoSMo, described in [10], could be used for a deformable image registration. A mean-squared error metric and a gradient descent optimizer were used for the registration process (Fig. 2).

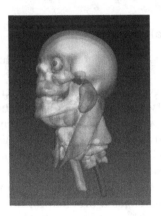

Fig. 2. CoSMo: Visualization of the mean model

2.3   CoSMo Adaptation

CoSMo is a model trained from clinically annotated data sets. Hereby, a statistical representation for every item of interest is obtained. For items with low variance, a rigid model item is trained, which is a probability map plus an average intensity image (for more in depth information see [9]). Structures with high variance are represented as deformable shape models. The model not only trains the possible deformations of the unique items, but how an item deforms, translates and rotates in correspondance to the other items and the complete model.

The adaptation step is divided into several levels. The structures which are best distinguishable within the data set are adapted first, while the structures with the lowest visible contrast, are adapted last. That way first, the model is initialized by locating the skull within the image data. Then, the bone structures are adapted. Next different muscles and glands, the eyes and the brain are adapted. And finally, the adaptation of the lymph node levels is executed. As output, a separate segmentation for each structure of the model is generated. For more in detail information on the process refer to [6].

2.4   Lymph Node Level Determination

The acquired lymph nodes in the CT image data and the segmented lymph node regions from CoSMo are finally combined to extract the lymph node levels of the sentinel lymph node and the active lymph nodes. To determine the lymph node level of a detected lymph node a nearest neighbour search with all lymph node levels retrieved from CoSMo is run. Since the SPECT activity for a lymph node sometimes only occupies one or two voxel within the image data, it might be possible that it does not directly overlap with a lymph node region but resides directly next to one. Therefore, the nearest neighbour algorithm was favored over an overlap metric.

As a result the clinician receives all lymph node levels with active nodes, that should be considered during the radiation therapy planning or surgical neck dissection.

3   Evaluation

The test setup for the evaluation was as follows. Three data sets from patients of Università degli studi di Parma (Italy) and four data sets from Clinique et Maternité Sainte-Elisabeth Namur (Belgium) were used. The data sets from the hospital in Italy consisted of a SPECT-CT and the data sets from the hospital in Belgium SPECT-CT and a radiation therapy planning CT. In addition, we received the information about the number of active nodes and their lymph node level from a clinical expert from each of the centers. This information was used as ground truth and was compared with the output of our algorithm. In total, 17 lymph nodes have been identified by the clinical experts within the 7 patient data sets. The goal was to detect these lymph nodes correctly in the CT data set and match them to their corresponding lymph node level. Table 1 represents the results of the evaluation. The second column contains the found structures. The third column lists how the found structures have been classified (either LN level 1–5 left/right or as an artifact). The last column lists the ground truth lymph node level obtained by a clinical expert. In addition Fig. 3 shows the result of such a detection.

For six out of seven patients all lymph nodes have been detected and located in the image data correctly. For patient 4 only one lymph node in Level II left was detected, although the clinical experts counted two. Visual inspection of the image data revealed, that the two lymph nodes are located extremly close to each other and the algorithm considers them as one lymph node. Although, this is not the desired output of the algorithm, it is negligible in clinical practice, because an active node has been located in this lymph node level. For radiation therapy or a neck dissection, the complete lymph node level is treated no matter if one or two lymph nodes have been detected. Three times, an activity was detected, that afterwards was correctly classified as an artifact. Only one lymph node was not classified accordingly (Patient 3 lymph node 3). The lymph node was considered as an artifact, although it was a retropharyngeal lymph node.

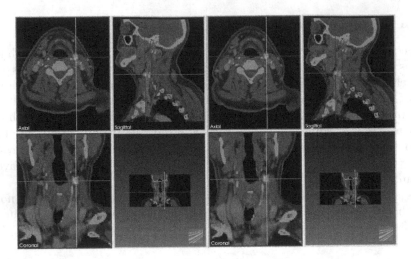

Fig. 3. Visualization of the second lymph node of patient 3 (left) and the overlay with lymph node level III left (right).

Table 1. Comparison of the detected active lymph node levels' with their ground truth

Patient #	Found lymph node #	Classified lymph node Level	Ground truth level
1	1 & 3	Level II left	Level II left (2 SLNs)
	2	Level II right	Level II right
	-	Artifact	-
2	1	Level II right	Level II right (1 SLN)
	2	Level II left	Level II left (1 SLN)
	-	Artifact	-
3	1	Level II left	Level II left (1 SLN)
	2	Level III left	Level III left(1 SLN)
	-	Artifact	Retropharyngeal
4	1	Level II left	Level II left (2 SLNs)
	2	Level II right	Level II right (1 SLN)
5	1	Level III left	Level III left (1 SLN)
	-	Artifact	-
	3	Level III right	Level III right (1 SLN)
6	1 & 3	Level III left	Level III left (2 SLNs)
	2	Level Ib left	Level Ib left (1 SLN)
7	1	Level II left	Level II left (1 SLN)
	2	Level III left	Level III left (1 SLN)

The reason for this misclassification is, that CoSMo only contains the lymph node level I - V left/right and not the Retropharyngeal area.

The runtime for the approach is the following. The duration for the SPECT detection is neglectable, it is around 1 s. CoSMo adaptation takes around 4 min and the SPECT-CT to CT registration takes around 1 min.

4   Conclusion

We have presented a novel approach to automatically extract additional information from SPECT-CT image data. The complete approach does not need any user interaction at all and can be run in background, before the image data is visually inspected by a clinical expert. The additional information obtained by our algorithm can be helpful in clinical practice for the planning of a surgical neck dissection or radiation therapy planning.

The algorithm has been evaluated on seven different patients and 17 lymph nodes have been inspected. 15 out of the 17 have been matched correctly. In one case two lymph nodes have been detected as one. In the other case the lymph node could not be matched properly because CoSMo currently does include the lymph node level (Retropharyngeal) in which the lymph node is located. As future work, additional lymph node levels could be included into CoSMo to match all needed lymph node levels. Finally, the approach has to be evaluated on a larger data set, to improve the statistical relevance of the evaluation result.

Recently, a new tracer has been presented, which primarily focuses on sentinel lymph nodes [1]. It rapidly clears out the tumor but remains in the lymph nodes. A consequence would be a better contrast for the nodes since the images would be free from the 'shine through effect'. This should greatly enhance the quality of the acquired data and thereby ease the processing by the algorithm. As a future work it would be very interesting, to acquire images with the new tracer and evaluate the approach on these.

In addition, it would be very interesting to evaluate if the proposed approach is suitable for PET imaging as well. Due to its similar nature, it should be feasible to use the algorithm on PET data as well, with some minor modifications.

The proposed algorithm is able to support radiation and surgical oncologists in their daily clinical routine. The approach features a fully automatic, fast and promising robust method to detect SLNs in the head and neck area and determine their corresponding lymph node levels.

Acknowledgements. This work is partially funded within the OraMod project (FP7-ICT-2013-10-611425) by the European Commission.

References

1. Agrawal, A., Civantos, F.J., Brumund, K.T., Chepeha, D.B., Hall, N.C., Carroll, W.R., Smith, R.B., Zitsch, R.P., Lee, W.T., Shnayder, Y., Cognetti, D.M., Pitman, K.T., King, D.W., Christman, L.A., Lai, S.Y.: [99mtc]tilmanocept accurately detects sentinel lymph nodes and predicts node pathology status in patients with oral squamous cell carcinoma of the head and neck: Results of a phase iii multi-institutional trial. Ann. Surg. Oncol. **22**(11), 3708–3715 (2015). doi:10.1245/s10434-015-4382-x

2. Atula, T., Shoaib, T., Ross, G.L., Gray, H.W., Soutar, D.S.: How many sentinel nodes should be harvested in oral squamous cell carcinoma? Eur. Arch. Oto-Rhino-Laryngol. **265**(1), 19–23 (2008). http://dx.doi.org/10.1007/s00405-007-0548-x

3. Daisne, J.F., Installé, J., Bihin, B., Laloux, M., Vander Borght, T., Mathieu, I., Lawson, G.: Spect/ct lymphoscintigraphy of sentinel node(s) for superselective prophylactic irradiation of the neck in cn0 head and neck cancer patients: a prospective phase i feasibility study. Radiat. Oncol. **9**(1), 121 (2014). http://dx.doi.org/10.1186/1748-717X-9-121

4. Dargent, D., Martin, X., Mathevet, P.: Laparoscopic assessment of the sentinel lymph node in early stage cervical cancer. Gynecol. Oncol. **79**(3), 411–415 (2000). http://www.sciencedirect.com/science/article/pii/S0090825800959997

5. D'Cruz, A.K., Vaish, R., Kapre, N., Dandekar, M., Gupta, S., Hawaldar, R., Agarwal, J.P., Pantvaidya, G., Chaukar, D., Deshmukh, A., Kane, S., Arya, S., Ghosh- Laskar, S., Chaturvedi, P., Pai, P., Nair, S., Nair, D., Badwe, R.: Elective versus therapeutic neck dissection in node-negative oral cancer. New Engl. J. Med. **373**(6), 521–529 (2015). doi:10.1056/NEJMoa1506007,pMID:26027881

6. Jung, F., Steger, S., Knapp, O., Noll, M., Wesarg, S.: COSMO - coupled shape model for radiation therapy planning of head and neck cancer. In: Linguraru, M.G., Oyarzun Laura, C., Shekhar, R., Wesarg, S., González Ballester, M.Á., Drechsler, K., Sato, Y., Erdt, M. (eds.) CLIP 2014. LNCS, vol. 8680, pp. 25–32. Springer, Cham (2014). doi:10.1007/978-3-319-13909-8_4

7. Lehmann, G.: Label object representation and manipulation with itk, August 2007. http://hdl.handle.net/1926/584

8. Patel, S.G., Shah, J.P.: TNM staging of cancers of the head and neck: striving for uniformity among diversity. CA: A Cancer J. Clin. **55**(4), 242–258 (2005). http://dx.doi.org/10.3322/canjclin.55.4.242

9. Steger, S., Jung, F., Wesarg, S.: Personalized articulated atlas with a dynamic adaptation strategy for bone segmentation in CT or CT/MR head and neck images (2014)

10. Steger, S., Kirschner, M., Wesarg, S.: Automated skeleton based multi-modal deformable registration of head & neck datasets. Med. Image Comput. Comput. Assist. Interv. MICCAI **2012**, 66–73 (2012)

11. Torre, L.A., Bray, F., Siegel, R.L., Ferlay, J., Lortet-Tieulent, J., Jemal, A.: Global cancer statistics, 2012. CA Cancer J. Clin. **65**(2), 87–108 (2015). http://dx.doi.org/10.3322/caac.21262

12. Yuen, A.P.W., Wei, W.I., Wong, Y.M., Tang, K.C.: Elective neck dissection versus observation in the treatment of early oral tongue carcinoma. Head Neck **19**(7), 583–588 (1997). http://dx.doi.org/10.1002/(SICI)1097-0347(199710)19:7⟨583::AID-HED4⟩3.0.CO;2-3

Towards an Automated Segmentation
of the Ventro-Intermediate Thalamic Nucleus

Elena Najdenovska[1,2(✉)], Constantin Tuleasca[3,4,5], João Jorge[1,6], José P. Marques[7],
Philippe Maeder[2], Jean-Philippe Thiran[2,4], Marc Levivier[3,5],
and Meritxell Bach Cuadra[1,2,4]

[1] Centre d'Imagerie BioMédicale (CIBM), University of Lausanne (UNIL), 1015 Lausanne,
Switzerland
elena.najdenovska@unil.ch
[2] Department of Radiology, Lausanne University Hospital (CHUV) and University of Lausanne
(UNIL), 1011 Lausanne, Switzerland
[3] Department of Clinical Neurosciences, Neurosurgery Service and Gamma Knife Center,
Lausanne University Hospital (CHUV), 1011 Lausanne, Switzerland
[4] Signal Processing Laboratory (LTS5), École Polytechnique Fédérale de Lausanne (EPFL),
1015 Lausanne, Switzerland
[5] Faculty of Biology and Medicine, University of Lausanne (UNIL), 1015 Lausanne, Switzerland
[6] Laboratory for Functional and Metabolic Imaging, École Polytechnique Fédérale de Lausanne
(EPFL), 1015 Lausanne, Switzerland
[7] Donders Center for Cognitive Neuroimaging, Radboud University,
6525 HP Nijmegen, The Netherlands

Abstract. The ventro-intermediate nucleus (Vim), as the others thalamic
subparts, cannot be directly visualized by current standard magnetic resonance
imaging (MRI), in daily clinical practice. Hence, for treatment of tremor in functional neurosurgery, where the commonly used target is the Vim, the targeting
procedure is done indirectly. We present a novel direct automated segmentation
of the Vim using only subject-related MRI information, specifically, diffusion
MRI at 3T and susceptibility weighted images (SWI) acquired at 7T. With a state-
of-the-art method based on local diffusion MR properties for automated subdivision of the thalamus, we first restrain the region of interest to the group of motor-
related nuclei. Then, this thalamic part is further subdivided, in graph parcellation
manner, using the intensity-related features provided by SWI together with prior
knowledge of the Vim localization inside the motor thalamic segment. Our
framework was tested in four healthy elderly subjects, for eight thalami in total,
and the results were evaluated by an experienced neurosurgeon, showing the
ability to directly detect the Vim area. The qualitative inspection indicated that
the proposed method outperforms standard multi-atlas based techniques.

Keywords: Vim · Automated segmentation · 7T susceptibility weighted images

M.J. Cardoso et al. (Eds.): CARE/CLIP 2017, LNCS 10550, pp. 141–150, 2017.
DOI: 10.1007/978-3-319-67543-5_14

1 Introduction

The ventro-intermediate nucleus (Vim) is part of the motor-group of thalamic nuclei. Its major importance comes from being the most common target in functional neuro-surgery as a treatment for tremor, either in standard procedures (deep brain stimulation or radiofrequency thalamotomy) or in alternative minimally invasive therapies (Vim radiosurgery or High Intensity Focused Ultrasound) [1, 2]. However, due to the lack of intrinsic or inherent contrast inside the thalamic area, the Vim is not directly visible on standard magnetic resonance imaging (MRI) routinely used in daily clinical practice acquired from field up to 3T. Consequently, the targeting for drug-resistant tremor is done in an indirect way by employing stereotactic coordinates or quadrilatere of Guiot [3]. Such approaches are mainly built upon a statistical average over the population and therefore, lack in representation of the individual variability.

To address these limitations, several research groups have made an attempt for an automated parcellation of the thalamus mainly based on diffusion-weighted images (DWI) acquired at 3T with the purpose of exploring the fibers orientation within the thalamic subparts [4–8]. In this context, Battistella et al. [4] recently proposed a robust method that partitions the thalamus in seven groups of nuclei using the Orientation Distribution Functions (ODFs) expressed in the Spherical Harmonic (SH) Basis that is outperforming the most advanced diffusion features so far. One of the segmented clusters represents the ventro-lateral ventral (VLV) thalamic part i.e. the motor-related group of nuclei including the Vim. However, the Vim cannot be accurately depicted with diffu-sion MRI, for instance as a separate component of VLV, mainly due to the relatively low spatial resolution of the standard DWI (~2 × 2 × 2 mm^3).

Advanced developments in MRI at ultra-high field (7T) provides not only better spatial resolution, but also an improved intensity-contrast variation inside the thalamus, namely with the susceptibility mapping approaches. Moreover, Abosch et al. have indi-cated the correspondence of the observed features on susceptibility-weighted imaging (SWI) acquired at 7T with the thalamic anatomy [9] and subsequently they suggested the possibility of a direct visualization of the Vim on those images. Nevertheless, while the subthalamic nucleus has been validated for 7T in a clinical frame, the Vim obser-vations remain purely descriptive.

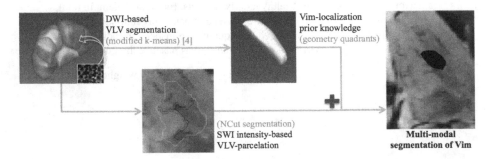

Fig. 1. Schematic overview of the proposed framework

The aim of this study is to automatically segment the Vim by combining SWI information at ultra-high field and prior knowledge of the VLV group of nuclei extracted from diffusion MRI. More specifically, we will combine NCut graph segmentation based on SWI intensity with a high-probability map of Vim localization derived from diffusion MRI thalamic clustering. Figure 1 shows a scheme of the proposed framework.

2   Materials and Methods

2.1   Dataset

The core of this study is performed in a dataset acquired at both 3 and 7T from four healthy elderly subjects (mean ± std: 67.2 ± 9.5 years, 3 males). Additional data from four healthy young subjects (28.5 ± 2.6 years, 2 males), for whom manual delineation of the Vim is available, was used for building atlases for comparison purposes. None of the subjects had any particular neurological disease nor a brain deformation caused by intracranial lesions. The study was approved by the local institutional review board and an informed consent was obtained from all the participants.

Image Acquisitions. The data from elderly subjects at 3T was acquired with a Prisma Siemens scanner and it included a T1-weighted (T1w, MPRAGE) sequence (TR/TE = 2300/2.03 ms, TI = 900 ms, voxel size: 1 mm^3) and DWI (64 gradient directions, b = 1000 s/mm^2, TR/TE = 7100/84 ms, voxel-size: 2.24 × 2.24 × 2.2 mm^3). T1w images from the healthy population were acquired with 3T TIM Trio Siemens scanner with similar acquisition parameters as those for the elderly population.

For all eight subjects, the ultra-high field data was acquired with a 7T, 68 cm-*wide bore* MRI system from SIEMENS Medical Solutions, equipped with a single-channel transmit/32-channel receive head RF array (Nova Medical). This data included axial SWI (with a restrained field of view, FoV, surrounding the thalamus, TR/TE = 28/20 ms, flip-angle 10°, voxel-size: 0.375 × 0.375 × 1 mm^3, 72 slices) and T1w (MP2RAGE) sequence (TR/TE = 6000/2.05 ms, TI$_1$/TI$_2$ = 800/2700 ms, flip-angles: 7/5°, voxel-size: 0.6 × 0.6 × 0.6 mm^3).

Common Image Space. We choose to work in the individual anterior commissure-posterior commissure (AC-PC) image space of each elderly subject. The image space was defined by the T1 template in MNI space of voxel size 0.5 × 0.5 × 0.5 mm^3 [10] whose AC-PC plane was aligned horizontally. Each 3T MPRAGE was transformed into this AC-PC space by a rigid transform, and the individual resulting image, *T1w_acpc*, was considered as reference for the successive image transformations described in the following sections.

2.2   Thalamic Parcellation

The preprocessing of the DWI included several steps: data denoising [11, 12], bias field [13, 14], motion [15] and eddy current corrections [16]. Furthermore, with a non-linear registration, using FSL's FNIRT [13], between the T1w_acpc and the respective fractional anisotropy (FA) map, we compensated the EPI distortions presented in the DWI data. On the preprocessed data we performed the Q-ball fitting of the Constant Solid Angle ODFs (FSL qboot) with maximum SH order of 6, accordingly to [4].

The thalamus masks were obtained from the FreeSurfer's subcortical parcellation, performed for each 3T MPRAGE, and further refined, as described in [4], by automatically removing voxels with FA value greater than 0.55 and celebro-spinal fluid's probability exceeding 5%. Subsequently to a qualitative comparison between the refined masks and the SWI where the thalamic borders appear more discernible, missing voxels were manually added mainly in the anterior and the lateral part of the inferior thalamic slices.

Following the framework description in [4], the thalamus was subdivided in 7 clusters while applying a modified k-means using as features the spatial position of the thalamic voxels and the corresponding ODF coefficients in the SH basis. The obtained results, including the VLV cluster were then brought in the AC-PC space by applying the non-linear transform, as described earlier, matching the FA and T1w_acpc image.

2.3   The Proposed Framework

The VLV cluster, other than Vim, includes several motor-related nuclei. However, in correspondence to the findings described in [9], in SW imaging, the ventral nuclei surrounding the Vim, such as ventro-caudalis (Vc) and ventro-odalis (Vo), appear as darker regions in comparison with our area of interest (see Fig. 2). These contrast differences we observed inside the VLV drove us to explore the SWI-intensity for a further VLV subdivision aiming towards an automated delineation of the Vim.

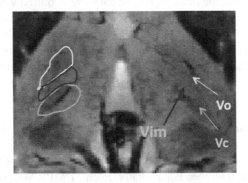

Fig. 2. Illsutration of the SWI visible structures surrounding the Vim in axial view. On the right side we have manually in-plane draw of the visible ventral nuclei in correspondence with the Schaltenbrand and Wahren atlas [17], while on the left they are indicated with arrows. The yellow represents the Vim, while the bright green and the bright orange ventro-caudalis (Vc) and ventro-odalis (Vo), which are surrounding the Vim as darker areas. (Color figure online)

SWI Preprocessing. The SWI images from our elderly cohort were corrected for intensity inhomogeneities using the N4ITK bias field correction algorithm [18]. The obtained images were first registered to the corresponding 7T MP2RAGE with a rigid transform and then brought to the AC-PC space by applying the analogous affine transform that matched the 7T MP2RAGE and T1w_acpc.

Primary analysis of the SWI data showed high intensity variability among the subjects and different head position in the scanner. Therefore, to standardize the image intensity appearing on these images, we applied the histogram equalization algorithm proposed by Nyul et al. [19] that represents an one-to-one image transformation and therefore, does not affect the image appearance. We work in a volume of interest (VOI) surrounding both thalami for each subject respectively. Figure 2 is representing an axial slice of the used VOI in one case. All four SWI images from the elderly population were used in the training step where the standard scale was build upon the deciles extracted from each image histogram. The results from this histogram matching are shown in Fig. 3.

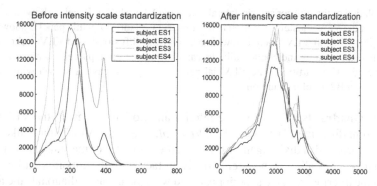

Fig. 3. Histogram equalization of the SWI intensity inside the thalamic area

To further enhance the edges and observable features on the SWI, the ITK gradient anisotropic diffusion filtering of conductance 0.3 was applied.

Graph Representation and Parcellation. The preprocessed SWI-intensity information inside the VLV was transformed in a graph representation of the data. More precisely, we constructed a k-nn graph with 50 nearest neighbors, where the edges' weights expressed the Gaussian weighting of the linear combination between the intensity distance (*Dint*) and the Euclidean distance among the VLV voxels (*Dpos*):

$$D = Dint + \gamma Dpos \tag{1}$$

where γ represents the ratio between *max(Dint)* and *max(Dpos)* and therefore, it acts as a scaling factor that brings the *Dpos* in the same range of values as *Dint*.

The parcellation of the graph was performed with Normalized Cut (NCut) partition [20]. We subdivided the VLV in 3 sub-clusters. The number 3 was chosen empirically since it gives a consistent parcellation pattern corresponding to our prior knowledge/hypothesis of the VLV structure: the region with bright SWI intensity as the expected one in the Vim area, the region with darker SWI intensity and an auxiliary part (see Fig. 4B1).

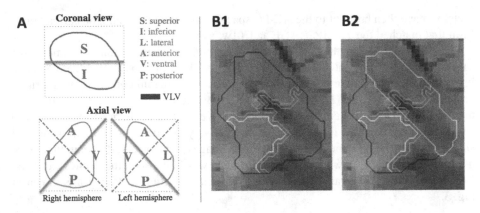

Fig. 4. Isolation of the inferior anterio-lateral part of the VLV cluster. Panel A shows a schematic illustration of the VLV-cluster separation in 8 geometrical quadrants, while panel B shows a real-case example of the left VLV in axial view. In panel B1 the diffusion-based VLV outline is given with the magenta contour and additionally we can observe the three parcels obtained from SWI intensity-based NCut partition. The VLV_ial part for the given case is shown with the white contour in panel B2. (Color figure online)

Geometry Quadrants. To isolate the inferior anterio-lateral part of the VLV cluster obtained from diffusion MRI (Sect. 2.2), *VLV_ial*, where the Vim is most likely to be found, we proceeded at dividing the VLV using the geometry of the smallest rectangular cuboid that contains all of its non-zero voxels. In fact, with the cuboid's mid-plane, we separated the inferior from the superior part and with the in-plane diagonals the anterio-lateral from the ventral-posterior part (see Fig. 4A).

The separated VLV_ial portion was used to confine the NCut parcellation to the expected localization of the Vim (Fig. 4B).

2.4 Multi-atlas Segmentation

In this work we propose a direct segmentation of the Vim by using subject specific information from both diffusion MRI and SWI. The state-of-the-art lacks in Vim-delineation approaches. However, if an atlas is available, this could be achieved with the atlas-based segmentation techniques. Hence, we additionally aim at performing a multi-atlas based segmentation and comparing it to the outcome of our multi-modal framework. As atlases we used SWI data from young subjects where the Vim was manually delineated by an experienced neurosurgeon. The manual delineation was mainly based upon the visible contrast variation together with the observation shown in [9] and the Schaltenbrand and Wahren atlas [17].

For transforming the atlases in each respective AC-PC space previously defined, our initial attempt was to directly match the SWIs but, presumably due to the variation of the FoV orientation among the subjects, all image registration technics failed to provide a good matching. Therefore, the atlases correspondence was done via the T1w images, by calculating consecutively linear and BSpline transform between the respective atlas' 3T MPRAGE and the T1w_acpc. The final multi-atlas outline was obtained by applying the Joint Label Fusion method with corrective learning [21] within the thalamic VOI previously defined.

3   Results

The proposed framework was tested for the group of elderly subjects or, more precisely, eight thalami in total. The intersection between the NCut parcellation and the VLV_ial portion mainly resulted in two subdivisions. Among the two, we choose as Vim outline the region showing brighter intensity (see Fig. 4 panel B). As described in Sect. 2.4, atlas-based segmentation using 4 thalami per hemisphere was also performed.

The multi-atlas outline represented in general smaller area than the multi-modal outline. However, overlap between both delimitations was always observed. Additionally, for six out of eight thalami, the major part of the multi-atlas Vim delimitation was inside the one from the multi-modal segmentation. For the remaining two cases, a blood vessel was observed in the targeted area disintegrating its intensity homogeneity (Fig. 5, right hemisphere of ES2 and ES4). Overall results are illustrated in Fig. 5.

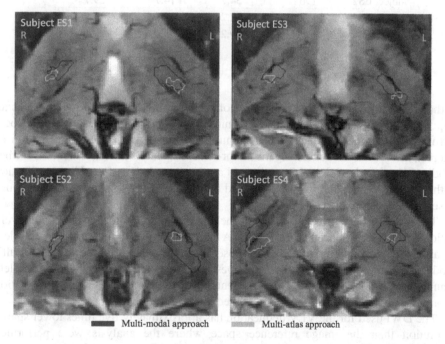

Fig. 5. Visual overview of the obtained findings for each tested subject respectively in an axial slice. The multi-modal outline corresponds to the violet contour, while the multi-atlas one to the green contour. (Color figure online)

The results provided by the proposed framework were qualitatively validated by the same neurosurgeon who did the manual delimitation of the Vim in the atlases. His observations were that, despite the tendency of the multi-modal approach to do a slight overestimation of the visually expected Vim extend by enclosing minor parts of the surrounding thalamic structures, they however portray more completely the region of interest than the small volumes provided by the multi-atlas approach. Additionally, the multi-modal delimitations are more consistent in symmetry over the hemispheres than the multi-atlas ones.

In the context of the size, the visual observations were confirmed with the calculated volumes of both multi-modal and multi-atlas segmentations given in Table 1. Since the expected size of the Vim is between 60 to 150 mm^3 [22], the volumes of the proposed multi-modal delimitation are sometimes marginally exceeding the expected range. In contrast to this, the multi-atlas delineations are importantly underestimating the size of the Vim.

Table 1. Volumes of the resulting Vim outlines

VOLUME [mm^3]	Multi-modal segmentation		Multi-atlas segmentation	
	Left	Right	Left	Right
Subject ES1	122.5	149.2	21.4	18.7
Subject ES2	196	54.7	14.7	29.7
Subject ES3	198.4	187.2	11.7	35
Subject ES4	176.1	129.2	5.4	29.1

4   Discussion

Although performed on a limited number of subjects, the present study represents an important step towards an automated segmentation of the Vim area. We used local diffusion MR properties inside the thalamus for delimitation of an initial region of interest, the VLV cluster enclosing the motor-related thalamic nuclei, which was further subdivided using the 7T SWI intensity and a prior knowledge of the Vim localization within the VLV. We additionally examined the ability of multi-atlas based techniques to segment the Vim.

The spatial distribution and extent of the resulting Vim outlines were qualitatively validated by an experienced neurosurgeon. A minor affinity of slightly imprecise borders regarding the surrounding structures was observed in the outcome of the proposed multi-modal method. Nevertheless, these outlines represent better and in more complete manner the Vim area than the limited extents provided by a multi-atlas segmentation approach. Analogue to this are the calculated volumes of the outlines.

The DWI used for the VLV delineation has approximately five times lower spatial resolution than the image reference space where the analysis were performed ($2.24 \times 2.24 \times 2.2$ mm^3 versus $0.5 \times 0.5 \times 0.5$ mm^3). As consequence we are prone to imprecise border delineation of the initial region of interest i.e. the VLV thalamic part. Another limitation comes from the non-robust contrast variation observed on the SWI together with the presence of the blood vessels in an indiscriminate mode, inside the VLV and the thalamus in general, increasing the potential of Vim's border inaccuracy. This could also have a major impact on direct visualization in some cases. Further studies should be done to understand the origin of the differences in feature appearance observed on SWI for the populations of different age. We believe that standardization of the SWI contrast could make this imaging method even more powerful tool for direct visualization, especially for direct targeting in functional neurosurgery in drug-resistant tremor.

In this study we have also shown that the imaging method based on the individual subjects' anatomy outperforms the approaches build from statistical average among a chosen population, such as the atlases. As limitation of the used multi-atlas approach we consider the image registration done between the respective T1w images on which the thalamus appears as a homogeneous area with borders that are difficult to discriminate. Hence, the information provided for the thalami matching and the corrective learning afterwards is not optimal. Possible improvement in this context could be the direct use of the SWI for the image matching procedure, since it provides much more features of the thalamic architecture. However, mainly due to the variation of the SWI FoV orientation, it was difficult to achieve such task in the presented data.

The proposed multi-modal framework should be further quantitatively evaluated against a manual delamination of the targeted area. Nevertheless, it represents a novel advancement in the field of automated subject-specific segmentation of the Vim.

Acknowledgements. The work was supported by the Swiss National Science Foundation (SNSF-205321-157040) and by the Centre d'Imagerie BioMédicale (CIBM) of the University of Lausanne (UNIL), the Swiss Federal Institute of Technology Lausanne (EPFL), the University of Geneva (UniGe), the Centre Hospitalier Universitaire Vaudois (CHUV), the Hôpitaux Universitaires de Genève (HUG), and the Leenaards and Jeantet Foundations.

References

1. Lipsman, N., Schwartz, M.L., Huang, Y., Lee, L., Sankar, T., Chapman, M., Hynynen, K., Lozano, A.M.: MR-guided focused ultrasound thalamotomy for essential tremor: a proof-of-concept study. Lancet Neurol. **12**, 462–468 (2013)
2. Witjas, T., Carron, R., Krack, P., Eusebio, A., Vaugoyeau, M., Hariz, M., Azulay, J.P., Regis, J.: A prospective single-blind study of Gamma Knife thalamotomy for tremor. Neurology **85**, 1562–1568 (2015)
3. Kondziolka, D., Ong, J.G., Lee, J.Y., Moore, R.Y., Flickinger, J.C., Lunsford, L.D.: Gamma Knife thalamotomy for essential tremor. J. Neurosurg. **108**, 111–117 (2008)
4. Battistella, G., Najdenovska, E., Maeder, P., Ghazaleh, N., Daducci, A., Thiran, J.P., Jacquemont, S., Tuleasca, C., Levivier, M., Bach Cuadra, M., Fornari, E.: Robust thalamic nuclei segmentation method based on local diffusion magnetic resonance properties. Brain Struct. Funct. (2016)
5. Behrens, T.E., Johansen-Berg, H., Woolrich, M.W., Smith, S.M., Wheeler-Kingshott, C.A., Boulby, P.A., Barker, G.J., Sillery, E.L., Sheehan, K., Ciccarelli, O., Thompson, A.J., Brady, J.M., Matthews, P.M.: Non-invasive mapping of connections between human thalamus and cortex using diffusion imaging. Nat. Neurosci. **6**, 750–757 (2003)
6. Mang, S.C., Busza, A., Reiterer, S., Grodd, W., Klose, A.U.: Thalamus segmentation based on the local diffusion direction: a group study. Magn. Reson. Med. **67**, 118–126 (2012). Official Journal of the Society of Magnetic Resonance in Medicine/Society of Magnetic Resonance in Medicine
7. Wiegell, M.R., Tuch, D.S., Larsson, H.B., Wedeen, V.J.: Automatic segmentation of thalamic nuclei from diffusion tensor magnetic resonance imaging. NeuroImage **19**, 391–401 (2003)

8. Ziyan, U., Tuch, D., Westin, C.-F.: Segmentation of thalamic nuclei from DTI using spectral clustering. In: Larsen, R., Nielsen, M., Sporring, J. (eds.) MICCAI 2006. LNCS, vol. 4191, pp. 807–814. Springer, Heidelberg (2006). doi:10.1007/11866763_99

9. Abosch, A., Yacoub, E., Ugurbil, K., Harel, N.: An assessment of current brain targets for deep brain stimulation surgery with susceptibility-weighted imaging at 7 tesla. Neurosurgery **67**, 1745–1756 (2010). Discussion 1756

10. Fonov, V.S., Evans, A.C., McKinstry, R.C., Almli, C.R., Collins, D.L.: Unbiased nonlinear average age-appropriate brain templates from birth to adulthood. NeuroImage **47**(Supplement 1), S102 (2009)

11. Tournier, J.D., Calamante, F., Connelly, A.: MRtrix: diffusion tractography in crossing fiber regions. Int. J. Imaging Syst. Technol. **22**, 53–66 (2012)

12. Veraart, J., Novikov, D.S., Christiaens, D., Ades-Aron, B., Sijbers, J., Fieremans, E.: Denoising of diffusion MRI using random matrix theory. NeuroImage **142**, 394–406 (2016)

13. Smith, S.M., Jenkinson, M., Woolrich, M.W., Beckmann, C.F., Behrens, T.E., Johansen-Berg, H., Bannister, P.R., De Luca, M., Drobnjak, I., Flitney, D.E., Niazy, R.K., Saunders, J., Vickers, J., Zhang, Y., De Stefano, N., Brady, J.M., Matthews, P.M.: Advances in functional and structural MR image analysis and implementation as FSL. NeuroImage **23**(Suppl 1), S208–S219 (2004)

14. Zhang, Y., Brady, M., Smith, S.: Segmentation of brain MR images through a hidden Markov random field model and the expectation-maximization algorithm. IEEE Trans. Med. Imaging **20**, 45–57 (2001)

15. Leemans, A., Jones, D.K.: The B-Matrix must be rotated when correcting for subject motion in DTI Data. Magn. Reson. Med. **61**, 1336–1349 (2009)

16. Andersson, J.L., Sotiropoulos, S.N.: An integrated approach to correction for off-resonance effects and subject movement in diffusion MR imaging. NeuroImage **125**, 1063–1078 (2016)

17. Schaltenbrand, G., Wahren, W.: Atlas for Stereotaxy of the Human Brain. Year Book Medical Publishers (1977)

18. Tustison, N.J., Avants, B.B., Cook, P.A., Zheng, Y.J., Egan, A., Yushkevich, P.A., Gee, J.C.: N4ITK: improved N3 bias correction. IEEE Trans. Med. Imaging **29**, 1310–1320 (2010)

19. Nyul, L.G., Udupa, J.K., Zhang, X.: New variants of a method of MRI scale standardization. IEEE Trans. Med. Imaging **19**, 143–150 (2000)

20. Shi, J.B., Malik, J.: Normalized cuts and image segmentation. In: Proceedings of CVPR IEEE, pp. 731–737 (1997)

21. Wang, H., Yushkevich, P.A.: Multi-atlas segmentation with joint label fusion and corrective learning-an open source implementation. Front. Neuroinform. **7**, 27 (2013)

22. Tuite, P.J., Dagher, A.: Magnetic Resonance Imaging in Movement Disorders: A Guide for Clinicians and Scientists. Cambridge University Press, Cambridge (2013)

Classification of Confocal Endomicroscopy Patterns for Diagnosis of Lung Cancer

Debora Gil[1], Oriol Ramos-Terrades[1], Elisa Minchole[2], Carles Sanchez[1(✉)],
Noelia Cubero de Frutos[2], Marta Diez-Ferrer[2], Rosa Maria Ortiz[2],
and Antoni Rosell[2]

[1] Computer Science Department, Computer Vision Center,
Universitat Autonoma de Barcelona,Barcelona, Spain
csanchez@cvc.uab.es
[2] Hospital de Bellvitge,Barcelona, Spain

Abstract. Confocal Laser Endomicroscopy (CLE) is an emerging imaging technique that allows the in-vivo acquisition of cell patterns of potentially malignant lesions. Such patterns could discriminate between inflammatory and neoplastic lesions and, thus, serve as a first in-vivo biopsy to discard cases that do not actually require a cell biopsy.

The goal of this work is to explore whether CLE images obtained during videobronchoscopy contain enough visual information to discriminate between benign and malign peripheral lesions for lung cancer diagnosis. To do so, we have performed a pilot comparative study with 12 patients (6 adenocarcinoma and 6 benign-inflammatory) using 2 different methods for CLE pattern analysis: visual analysis by 3 experts and a novel methodology that uses graph methods to find patterns in pretrained feature spaces. Our preliminary results indicate that although visual analysis can only achieve a 60.2% of accuracy, the accuracy of the proposed unsupervised image pattern classification raises to 84.6%.

We conclude that CLE images visual information allow in-vivo detection of neoplastic lesions and graph structural analysis applied to deep-learning feature spaces can achieve competitive results.

1 Introduction

Incidence of Solitary Pulmonary Nodule (SPN) is increasing, but its diagnose can be challenging, especially when it is located in the periphery. Bronchoscopy is a minimally invasive procedure used in the diagnosis of central airways and lung tissue pathologies. Nowadays, new bronchoscopic procedures such as endobronchial ultrasound, ultrathin bronchoscopy guided by fluoroscopy or electromagnetic navigation, where a combination of endoscopic and radiological images are used, have increased bronchoscopy diagnostic yield.

Confocal laser endomicroscopy (CLE) is a new technique that can be combined with bronchoscopy to provide images of cells. CLE is a probe containing optic fibres that is introduced through the channel within the bronchoscope. Once CLE is in touch with the airways wall (proximal or distal airways) it will

© Springer International Publishing AG 2017
M.J. Cardoso et al. (Eds.): CARE/CLIP 2017, LNCS 10550, pp. 151–159, 2017.
DOI: 10.1007/978-3-319-67543-5_15

show microscopic images of lung tissue [1]. Up to now, CLE has been mainly used in gastrointestinal endoscopy to detect changes in mucosa and cellular patterns for in-vivo classification of neoplastic and inflammatory lesions in colon cancer diagnosis [1–3]. Only in recent studies, CLE using fluorescence has been applied to the visualization of lung structures (alveolar ducts and bronchial microstructures) [4, 5]. In particular there are 2 works describing the visual characteristics of neoplastic cellular patterns observed in CLE.

In [6], the authors analyzed the patterns observed in CLE images from 12 patients with nodules in main airways. In that study, the visual patterns for 3 different types of cancerous lesions were described and compared to the visual appearance of normal mucosa. The main conclusion of that work is that the distribution and size of cell nuclei is more heterogeneous and sparse for malign nodules. The other study reports about cellular patterns of CLE with methylene blue dye taken from peripheral lesions of 3 patients [7]. In that work the authors also conclude that the technique might allow in-vivo assessment of solitary peripheral nodules during the bronchoscopic exploration. Although clinical studies indicate that CLE images of the lung could provide enough visual information to differentiate between malign and benign cellular patterns, as far as we known, there are no studies assessing CLE visual patterns in an quantitative systematic way. The goal of this work is to characterize cellular patterns in CLE images of peripheral lung nodules and assess their potential to discriminate between malign and benign lesions.

A main challenge in the development of image processing and classification methods for emerging medical imaging technologies is the limited amount of data available to design, train and test the decision support system. Such a condition has a negative impact in state-of-art classification methods that demand huge amounts of annotated data to achieve accurate and reliable results, such as Support Vector Machines (SVM) [8] and more recently deep learning algorithms [9].

Alternatives to supervised classification methods are either retrieval systems or unsupervised clustering algorithms. Both approaches rely on a similarity measure defined in the image feature space to either retrieve annotated cases similar to an unknown input image or group images presenting similar visual features. In fact, the only work addressing assessment of cellular patterns in CLE proposes a content-based image retrieval system based on Bag of Words and k-nearest neighbour (kNN) clustering [2]. Although, the use of such software restricts to classification of CLE patterns in gastrointestinal endoscopic procedures its 89.6% of accuracy proves the potential of unsupervised methods to achieve clinically meaningful conclusions in case of a low number of samples.

We present a novel approach to find patterns in visual feature spaces by exploring the space topological structure. In order to extract topology, proximity relationships among a set of discrete samples is codified using a graph representation. The open sets defining the topology correspond to subgraphs fulfilling some connectivity criterion. To compute such subgraphs, we use community detection methods from social network analysis. Finally, the profile computed using the annotated samples, belonging to each community that a CLE image belongs to, defines the diagnose of non-annotated cases. The preliminary results obtained for 171 images with malign and benign patterns achieve a 84.6% of overall accuracy and a 81.1% of recall in cancer detection.

2   Classification of Confocal Patterns

Our approach consists in constructing a graph representation of CLE images based on visual features and try to discover potentially overlapping groups of images that share common properties. We refer to such groups as communities borrowing the terminology from the social network community. The rational of this approach is the following. Given a network of images (users) connected by means of visual appearance, we apply community detection algorithms to infer group of images that share similar properties. The annotations (clinical data in our case) made on the community images allow the definition of a community profile that can be assigned to images in the community without annotations. Since a CLE image can belong to more than one community we have to merge the community profiles it belongs to. In this section we describe all the main steps of our method: construction of the graph codifying feature space connectivity, graph community detection representing space topology and definition of profile (diagnosis in our case) for non-annotated images (see Fig. 1).

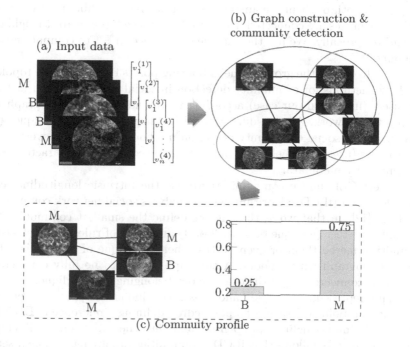

Fig. 1. Construction of CLE image clusters: (a) original images and feature vectors, (b) graph construction and community detection and (c) community profile.

The topology of a space is given by a collection of open subsets that cover the whole space [10]. Such collection defines, for each point of the space, a set of neighbouring points given by all points included in the subsets the point belongs to. Conversely, the set of neighbours of each point defines a topology in the space. Although unsupervised clustering is also based on neighbourhoods, a main difference with a topological approach is the criterion used to compute the open sets. In most unsupervised clustering such neighbourhoods are defined using a metric on the Euclidean space given by feature vectors. In a metric space, the collection of open sets are "balls" (points at equal distance to a given point). Since all open sets have equal dimension and shape, the resulting topology is very rigid in the sense that might have limited capability to describe clusters with complex structures of different dimensions.

The first step to obtain a topology is to represent the proximity among feature points. In the discrete domain, the spatial proximity of a set of points (images), sampled in a feature space, can be represented using an undirected graph, being the nodes the feature points representing images and being the edges defined according to similarity measure, or *friendship*, among neighbouring images. In the context of social networks, most applications (like Facebook or Tinder) grant connection between two users in case that they have mutually accepted a friendship request. An equivalent criterion on a image network is to use the mutual-kNN to define the connectivity of the graph [11]. The mutual-kNN criterion connects two images, I_i and I_j, if their feature points, $x_i \in \mathbb{R}^n$ and $x_j \in \mathbb{R}^n$, both of them are among the k-th nearest neighbours of the other. That is, two images are connected if x_i is ranked on the top k nearest neighbours of x_j and reciprocally. We use the Euclidean distance in $\mathbb{R}^n$ to compute nearest neighbours.

In order to obtain the groups of neighbouring points that define the topology, we will use methods for community detection in social networks. Such methods group users (images in our case) according to the adjacency of the graph representing the network. A main difference with other clustering techniques (like k-means) is that social community detection methods allow group overlapping. So that nodes (users) can belong to more than one community, characterized by each community metadata.

To detect CLE image communities we use the intrinsic longitudinal community detection (iLCD) algorithm, which analyses social network communities along time [12]. In that work, the authors define the smallest community that they want to detect (a clique of order 3 or 4) and a set of rules that detect new communities, merge them or even destroy them. A clique of order c is a fully connected subgraph with c nodes. A subgraph is said to be fully connected if each node is connected to all the other nodes belonging to the clique.

A clique represents a simplex and it is a continuous mapping (homeomorphism) into a topological space of a polyhedron defining a reference in Euclidean space [10]. A simplex defines an open set and thus the collection of all simplex define a topology. It follows that iLCD communities are giving the open sets of a topology defined by simplicial complexes, so we can describe richer geometries of our feature space.

The last step of our method is to take advantage of the above geometric representation to compute CLE image profiles for clinical diagnosis purposes. The profile of a non-annotated image is given by the fusion of the community profiles, in which it belongs to. Given that in this work we face a 2-class problem, we use the argmax criterion on the diagnosed: malign or benign cases, and therefore assign the most frequent label to the new image.

3 Experiments

3.1 Experimental Set-Up

A total of 12 patients (cases) from Hospital Universitari de Bellvitge with SPN or lung mass referred for bronchoscopy were included in the study. In the end, 6 patients had adenocarcinoma and 6 patients showed benign inflammatory changes. CLE images were obtained using a flexible bronchoscope BF-160, Olympus and a Alveloflex-Cellvizio (Manua Kea Technologies) 660 nm miniprobe for acquisition of CLE images. Virtual bronchoscopy using Lung Point was used to plan the path to the lesions. Methylene blue dye was used to enhance cellular pattern.

For each case, 2–6 video sequences lasting between 1–2.5 min each were acquired and processed with Cellvizio Viewer to enhance the blue channel. Video sequences were visually explored to select the between 10 and 15 images presenting a clear cellular pattern. In total, we collected 162 images, 78 from adenocarcinoma and 79 from inflammation. Figure 2 shows 3 images from each group. Cells nuclei correspond to brilliant spots in images. We note that for benign-inflammatory images, their distribution and size is homogeneous. Meanwhile malignant patterns are characterized by a clustering of cells that results in an overall heterogeneous appearance of images which have areas of low fluorescence.

Although any feature extraction technique can be applied, we have chosen a visual descriptor coming from deep learning architectures since they are proving to outperform handcraft descriptors in many computer vision applications. We used the VGG Convolutional Neural Network (CNN), which was trained on the ImageNet 1,000 object categories [13]. This CNN computes a global image descriptor obtained as the concatenation of the activation values of the last CNN convolution layer, and just before the fully connected layers which classify the 1,000 objects. This layer gives us a 4096-dimensional real-valued vector that we reduce using principal component analysis to 100 dimensions, which roughly represent the 90% of the energy the VGG vector.

We have compared our method to k-means and to kNN to assess the performance of the propose method in different aspects. The accuracy of k-means will indicate the discriminative power of VGG features, while comparison to kNN will show the differences between a description of clusters based on topology like ours and a standard metric approach. We assign to each cluster the most frequent label of the images belonging to it. We compare the value of such label to each image diagnosis to compute recall each class (malign, benign) and overall classification accuracy.

Concerning algorithm parameter settings, we applied all methods using different parameter configurations and we selected the best performer for comparisons. The numbers reported in Sect. 3.2 were obtained with graphs constructed using $k = 10$, $k = 18$ clusters for k-means and $k = 20$ for kNN.

Finally, images were shown to 3 expert observers who ignore the histopathological diagnosis for a blind visual labelling. Recall for each class and overall accuracy were computed for each expert. Aside, 2 of the observers were asked to provide a diagnosis for each patient based on the visual inspection of the whole set of images to assess accuracy in their final diagnosis.

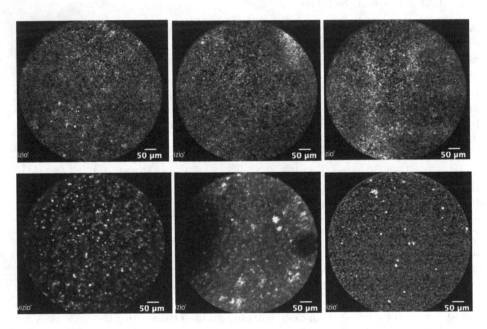

Fig. 2. Examples of CLE images for benign-inflammatory (top images) and malign-adenocarcinoma (bottom images) cases.

3.2   Results

The overall average accuracy in classification achieved by visual inspection of images was only 60.2% and presented a large variability among experts and cases. For malign images, recall was 72.8% in average with values per each observer equal to 84.2% for observer 1, 63.2% for observer 2 and 71.1% for observer 3. Benign images had even more variability with recall equal to 36.1% for observer 1, 51.2% for observer 2 and 60.5% for observer 3 and an average recall 49.2%. Results for visual classification are summarized for each case in Table 1 with benign cases indicated with (B) and malign ones with (M). Concerning accuracy

Table 1. Analysis of CLE images done by 3 observers.

	Case 1 (M)	Case 2 (B)	Case 3 (M)	Case 4 (B)	Case 5 (M)	Case 6 (B)	Case 7 (B)	Case 8 (M)	Case 9 (M)	Case 10 (M)	Case 11 (B)	Case 12 (B)
Obs. 1	7/7	2/15	9/15	5/15	13/13	6/14	4/12	12/12	14/14	9/15	7/15	7/15
Obs. 2	6/7	11/15	4/15	7/15	13/13	7/14	3/12	10/12	13/14	2/15	2/15	14/15
Obs. 3	5/7	12/15	5/15	6/15	11/13	9/14	4/12	10/12	14/14	9/15	9/15	12/15
AA	85.7%	55.5%	40.0%	40.0%	94.8%	52.3%	30.5%	88.8%	97.6%	44.4%	40.0%	73.3%

in final diagnosis, both experts issued the right diagnosis in 7/12 cases (66.6%), made a bad decision in 3/12 and did not agree in 2/12.

The overall accuracy for the proposed method (labelled GraphCom from now on) is 84.6%, 81.3% for kNN and 82.4% for k-means. Recall for malign images is 88.1% for GraphCom, 84.5% for kNN and 78.6% for k-means, while for benign cases recall is 81.2% for GraphCom, 78.2% for kNN and 86.2% for k-means. Results for each case reported in Table 2 show a lower variability than visual assessment. It is worth noticing that in case that final diagnosis was given by the most frequent label in each case, GraphCom would issue the right diagnosis in 12/12 cases (100%), kNN in 11/12 (91.6%) and k-means in 10/12 cases (83.3%). For both, kNN and k-means the wrong diagnosis were for malignant cases, which implies cancer detection rate equal to 83.3% for kNN and 66.6% for k-means.

Table 2. Analysis of CLE images done by the 3 unsupervised methods.

	Case 1 (M)	Case 2 (B)	Case 3 (M)	Case 4 (B)	Case 5 (M)	Case 6 (B)	Case 7 (B)	Case 8 (M)	Case 9 (M)	Case 10 (M)	Case 11 (B)	Case 12 (B)
GraphCom	7/7	14/15	9/15	14/15	11/13	13/14	12/12	7/12	11/14	12/15	15/15	10/15
kNN	7/7	13/15	10/15	12/15	11/13	14/14	12/12	7/12	7/14	12/15	15/15	10/15
k-means	7/7	12/15	14/15	12/15	10/13	14/14	12/12	5/12	7/14	14/15	15/15	11/15

4 Conclusions

The goal of this work was to determine whether CLE with methylene blue could potentially be useful to assess peripheral SPN. To do so, a pilot study with 12 patients (6 adenocarcinoma, 6 benign) and 171 images was conducted. Two main conclusions can be derived from our pilot study.

A first disappointing conclusion is that visual analysis by several individuals of CLE images looking for differences between neoplastic and inflammatory diseases showed an important inter and intra observer bias. In addition, identifying differences between malignancy and non-malignancy by visual inspection can be challenging given the similarities between both confocal patterns. Looking at our results, visual inspection is not enough to give a diagnosis of malignancy versus benign pathologies base on CLE images, with only 60% and 66% average accuracy between 2 and 3 observers respectively.

The good news is that image analysis can obtain enough information from CLE to discriminate between inflammatory and cancerous patterns using non-supervised techniques. The discriminative power of VGG features (given by k-means clustering) is quite high with a 82.4% of overall accuracy. However recall for malign cases drops to 78.6% and accuracy in final diagnosis is 83.3% overall but only a 66.6 in case of adenocarcinoma. In this paper, we have proposed to use a graph representation of the feature space combined with community detection algorithms. Our method provides a more flexible description of the feature space topology that increases accuracy in malign patterns to 88.1% and reaches a 100% in final diagnosis.

In summary, our preliminary results indicate that CLE images contain enough visual information for in-vivo detection of neoplastic lesions that could be extracted using graph structural analysis. The promising results obtained in this pilot study, encourage further research on community detection and graph structural methods as tools to design diagnosis support systems able to reach clinically meaningful conclusions with scarce annotated data.

Acknowledgments. Work supported by projects DPI2015-65286-R, FIS-ETES PI09/90917, 2014-SGR-1470 and Fundació Marató TV3 20133510. Also supported by CERCA Programme/Generalitat de Catalunya. The Titan X Pascal used for this research was donated by the NVIDIA Corporation. Finally, Debora Gil is supported by the Serra Hunter Program.

References

1. Jabbour, J.M., Saldua, M.A., Bixler, J.N., Maitland, K.C.: Confocal endomicroscopy: instrumentation and medical applications. Ann. Biomed. Eng. **40**(2), 378–397 (2012)
2. André, B., Vercauteren, T., Buchner, A.M., et al.: Software for automated classification of probe-based confocal laser endomicroscopy videos of colorectal polyps. World J. Gastroenterol. **18**(39), 5560–5569 (2012)
3. Sanduleanu, S., Driessen, A., Gomez-Garcia, E., Hameeteman, W., de Brune, A., Masclee, A.: In vivo diagnosis and classification of colorectal neoplasia by chromoendoscopy guided confocal laser endomicroscopy. Clin. Gastroenterol. Hepatol. **8**, 371–378 (2010)
4. Thiberville, L., Salaun, M., Lachkar, S., Dominique, S., Moreno-Swirc, S., Vever-Bizet, C., Bourg-Heckly, G.: Human in vivo fluorescence microimaging of the alveolar ducts and sacs during bronchoscopy. Eur. Respir. J. **33**, 974–985 (2009)
5. Fuchs, F., Zirlik, S., Hildner, K.: Fluorescein-aided confocal laser endomicroscopy of the lung. Respiration **81**, 32–38 (2010)
6. Fuchs, F., Zirlik, S., Hildner, K., Schubert, J., Vieth, M., Neurath, M.: Confocal laser endomicroscopy for diagnosing lung cancer in vivo. Eur. Respir. J. **41**, 1401–1408 (2013)
7. Hassan, T., Piton, N., Lachkar, S., Salan, M., Thiberville, L.: A novel method for in vivo imaging of solitary lung nodules using navigational bronchoscopy and confocal laser microendoscopy. Lung **193**(5), 773–778 (2015)
8. Burges, C.J.C.: A tutorial on support vector machines for pattern recognition. Data Min. Knowl. Discov. **2**(2), 121–167 (1998)

9. Bengio, Y.: Learning deep architectures for AI. Found. Trends Mach. Learn. **2**(1), 1–127 (2009)
10. Greenberg, M.J., Harper, J.R.: Algebraic Topology: A First Course. Addison-Wesley, Redwood City (1981)
11. Luo, Q., Zhang, S., Huang, T., Gao, W., Tian, Q.: Superimage: packing semantic-relevant images for indexing and retrieval. In: ICMR (2014)
12. Cazabet, R., Amblard, F., Hanachi, C.: Detection of overlapping communities in dynamical social networks. In: ICSC, pp. 309–314 (2010)
13. Chatfield, K., Simonyan, K., Vedaldi, A., Zisserman, A.: Return of the devil in the details: delving deep into convolutional nets. In: BMVC (2014)

Automated Classification for Breast Cancer Histopathology Images: Is Stain Normalization Important?

Vibha Gupta[1]([⊠]), Apurva Singh[2], Kartikeya Sharma[3], and Arnav Bhavsar[1]

[1] Indian Institute of Technology Mandi, Mandi, India
vibha_gupta@students.iitmandi.ac.in, arnav@iitmandi.ac.in
[2] Manipal Institute of Technology, Manipal, India
apurva1095@gmail.com
[3] National Institute of Technology Hamirpur, Hamirpur, India
09kartikeya@gmail.com

Abstract. Breast cancer is one of the most commonly diagnosed cancer in women worldwide. A popular diagnostic method involves histopathological microscopy imaging, which can be augmented by automated image analysis. In histopathology image analysis, stain normalization is an important procedure of color transfer between a source (reference) and the test image, that helps in addressing an important concern of stain color variation. In this work, we hypothesize that if color-texture information is well captured with suitable features using data containing sufficient color variation, it may obviate the need for stain normalization.

Considering that such an image analysis study is relatively less explored, some questions are yet unresolved such as (a) How can texture and color information be effectively extracted and used for classification so as to reduce the burden on the uniform staining or stain normalization. (b) Are there good feature-classifier combinations which work consistently across all magnifications? (c) Can there be an automated way to select reference image for stain normalization?

In this work, we attempt to address such questions. In the process, we compare the independent texture and color channel information with that of some more sophisticated features which consider jointly color-texture information. We have extracted above features using images with and without stain normalization to validate the above hypothesis. Moreover, we also compare different types of contemporary classification in conjunction with the above features. Based on the results of our exhaustive experimentation we provide some useful indications.

Keywords: Histopathology image analysis · Stain normalization · Color-texture features · SVM · Random forest

1 Introduction

Breast cancer is the most common cancer in women worldwide and is the second leading cause of cancer deaths in women, after lung cancer [1]. One of the

© Springer International Publishing AG 2017
M.J. Cardoso et al. (Eds.): CARE/CLIP 2017, LNCS 10550, pp. 160–169, 2017.
DOI: 10.1007/978-3-319-67543-5_16

common approaches used for cancer detection is histopathology; it is defined as the microscopic examination of the histological sections of a biopsy sample by a pathologist in order to study the effects of a particular disease. Computer-aided approaches with image analysis and machine learning can be included in digital pathology to achieve quick and reproducible results. Computer aided diagnostic (CAD) models are also important as they assist pathologists in locating and identifying abnormalities in the breast tissue images.

A concern in histopathology image based assessment is the variation in color is obtained due to a number of factors like chemical reactivity from different manufacturers, differences in color responses of slide scanners or due to the light transmission being a function of slide thickness. However, this variability only partially limits the interpretation of images by pathologists. But leads to a large variation in the efficiency of automated image analysis algorithms. This problem can be partially reduced by incorporating the use of standardized staining protocols and automated staining machines. Stain normalization algorithms [2–4] have also been recently introduced to address stain variation, with the aim of matching stain colors of whole slide image with a given template.

One of the naive options to deal with color constancy is to convert color image to grayscale. In [5] author extracted features from a grayscale version of a query image. Conversion of an image into grayscale gives us the average of concentrations of the tissue components and does not tell us the relative amounts of each of them. Further, this also does not make effective use of the color information which is present. Recent research in histopathology has confirmed that color information is quite significant in quantitative analysis.

The outstanding ability of a pathologist to identify stain components is not only due to the utilization of color information but also because of incorporating the spatial dependency of tissue structures. The use of standardized staining protocols and automated staining machines may improve staining quality by yielding a more accurate and consistent staining. However, eliminating all the underlying sources of variation is infeasible.

Indeed, methods that investigate the importance of staining in conjunction with classification framework have also been developed. In [6], authors investigate the importance of stain normalization in tissue classification utilizing convolution network. In the same way, the authors in [7] perform the classification of prostate tumor regions via stain normalization and adaptive cell density estimation. On the other hand, there also exists some work which considers the utilization of color information without the use of stain normalization. The works in [8] and [9] propose the use color information in addition to texture. Milagro et al. [8] propose the combinations of traditional texture features and color spaces. Furthermore, they have also considered different classifiers such as Adaboost learning, bagging trees, random forest, Fisher discriminant and SVM. In [9], authors utilized color and differential invariants to assign class posterior probabilities to pixels and then perform a probabilistic classification.

The above approaches suggest different views about the consideration of stain normalization for classification. Inspired by this, our primary contribution in the

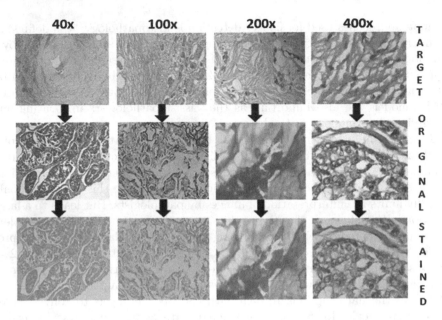

Fig. 1. Reference images chosen for normalization (top), sample of original images (middle), and obtained stain normalized images using the target images (bottom)

present work, is to explicitly provide indications towards addressing the question about how important is stain normalization for automatic classification, and whether there may exist useful features which inherently capture the color-texture variability without performing stain normalization. In other words, we attempt to justify the role of color-texture information in automated classification framework without performing stain normalization. We believe that such a study is important from a systems perspective, as it may help reduce the stain normalization overhead for automated histopathology classification systems. We note that such an indication of mitigating the need for stain normalization assumes that the training data contains images with different stain color/intensity, that helps in capturing the color-texture variability. We validate this hypothesis on a reasonably large dataset containing such images.

In this primary context, our work also has the following salient contributions about methodology and evaluation: (1) Exploring joint color-texture features and various contemporary classifiers, which makes the proposed work also serve as an extended comparative review. (2) Suggesting an automatic approach to select the reference (target) image for stain normalization where it is not available. Figure 1 shows examples of stained images of each magnification generated using target images. (3) Demonstrating an improved performance of the proposed method with joint color-texture features with respect to the state-of-the-art.

2 Proposed Approach

We now discuss the overall framework of proposed approach including: dataset description, stain normalization, feature descriptors, and contemporary classifiers. Due to lack of space, we briefly describe the features and classifiers with suitable references. Figure 3 depicts our overall framework.

2.1 Dataset Description

In this work, we use BreakHis dataset [10] that contains fairly large amount of histopathology images (7909). A detailed description is provided in Table 3.

In [10–12], authors developed the framework to classify breast cancer histopathological images utilizing the BreakHis dataset. In [10], a series of experiments utilizing six different state-of-art texture descriptors such as Local Binary Pattern (LBP), Completed Local Binary Pattern (CLBP), Threshold Adjancey Statistics (PFTAS), Grey-Level Co-occurrence Matrix (GLM), Local Phase Quantization (LPQ), Oriented FAST and rotated BRIEF (ORB), and four different classifiers were evaluated and showed the accuracy at patient level. In [11], Alexnet [13] was used for extracting features and classification. Bayramoglu et al. [12] proposed a magnification independent model utilizing deep learning to classify the benign and malignant cases. The magnification independent system is trained with images of different magnifications, and thus can handle the scale diversity in microscopic images.

2.2 Stain Normalization Procedure

Various methods [2–4] have been developed to automate the standardization process of histopathological images to reduce the effect of variation that exists in staining protocol. In [2] authors utilized chromatic and density distributions for each individual stain class in the hue-saturation-density (HSD) color model i.e. the spatial dependency of tissue structures was incorporated along with color information. In experiments, the target template was chosen based on opinion of two pathologists, who studied a large number of slides from two different laboratory. The high contrast between hematoxylin and eosin staining (H & E) and visibility of the nuclear texture were taken into consideration while choosing template image. In [3], the authors use the linear transform in a perceptual color space for matching the color distribution of an image to that of a target image. In [4], authors also utilized pathologist-preferred target image to generate structure-preserving color normalization. These stain normalization methods require prior knowledge of reference stain vectors for every dye present in the histopathogical images.

Due to the unavailability of a target template in the public dataset used in this work, we automatically select the target image from the dataset. Our approach considers that the target stain chromatic information should be considered that which occurs most commonly, so that a large number of images need not be color-transformed. Thus, we suggest the following process: (1) First, all the images in dataset are converted from RGB color-space to HSV color-space.

(2) We choose H and S component for further analysis as Hue and Saturation essentially relate to the chromatic information. (3) A K-means clustering algorithm is applied to form the desired number of clusters. The number of clusters chosen is the double of the number of different Hue that are found on manual examination of different images. This is to ensure that we have a good enough separation of images of different Hue. (4) The number of stain hues in the dataset found after manual examination are five. So we chose to create 10 clusters. In the pictorial representation of Fig. 2, we show less number of clusters for better clarity. (5) We choose the cluster that has highest number of images. In this cluster we find out the mean H and S value of image which is the closest to the centroid of the cluster using Euclidean distance measure. The corresponding image is used as the target image after conversion to RGB color-space.

The proposed procedure is applied separately to images of different magnifications. At the end, we have one target image for each magnification group of images. After selecting target image, we use stain normalization method proposed by [3] to normalize the dataset. Figure 2 illustrates the overall procedure for selecting target image. Figure 2 is just a way to depict the procedure and is not a real picture of our plots.

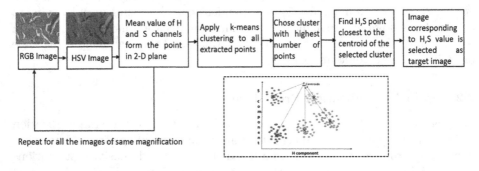

Fig. 2. Selection of target image.

2.3   Feature Descriptors and Contemporary Classifiers

Various texture features that consider the mutual dependency of color channel as well as the features that don't utilize the color information are extracted in order to support believe that we have made. Due to space constraint we are not providing the detailing of features. Gray level co-occurence matrix (GLCM), Completed local binary pattern (CLBP) [14], and Local phase quantization (LPQ) [15] are used to extract plain texture. For capturing joint color-texture variability, features such as Opponent Colour Local Binary pattern (OCLBP) [16], Gabor features on Gaussian color model [17], Multilayer Coordinate Clusters representation (MCCR) [18], and Parameter-free Threshold Adjacency Statistics (PFTAS) [19] are utilized. Note that the choice of features and classifiers is simply based on the popularity of the traditional texutre features, and considering some recently reported color-texture features.

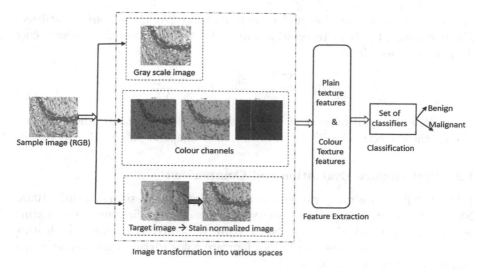

Fig. 3. Overall process of image classification.

Various contemporary classifiers [20] such as Support Vector Machine (SVM), Nearest Neighbors (NN) and Random forest (RF) are experimented with above listed texture features. For the proposed study, we utilize following variants of mentioned classifiers: (1) Liner SVM: Linear kernel, (2) Gaussian SVM: RBF kernel and kernel scale set to $2\sqrt{P}$, (3) K-NN: 100 neighbors and euclidean metric for distance measure, (4) RF: number of trees (30), maximum number of splits (20). Thus, the study also serves as a comparative review of performance for the above mentioned features and classifiers for the considered problem.

Figure 3 illustrates the overall structure utilized for the proposed study. As indicated earlier, the primary intention of this study is to consider the effect of stain normalization for automated breast cancer histopathology image classification. Thus, we test the classification performance with gray-scale image, stain normalized images, and original non-normalized images.

3 Results and Discussion

3.1 Training-Testing Protocol and Evaluation Metric

In our experiments, we have randomly chosen 58 patients (70%) for training and remaining 25 for testing (30%). This also enables fair comparison with a state-of-the-art approach [10–12]. We train the above listed contemporary classifiers using images for the chosen 58 patients, and have also used five trials of random selection of training-testing data. These trained models are tested using images of the remaining images 25 patients.

To compare the results with existing approach [10–12], we use patient recognition rate (PRR) as evaluation metric. However, some other evaluation metrics such as recall, precision, area under the ROC curve (AUC) can also be utilized. The definition of patient recognition rate (PRR), which uses the patient score (PS), is given as follows:

$$PRR = \frac{\sum_{i=1}^{N} PS_i}{N} \quad PS = \frac{N_{rec}}{N_P} \tag{1}$$

where N is the total number of patients (available for testing), and N_{rec} and N_P are the correctly classified and total cancer image of patient P respectively.

3.2   Performance Evaluation and Comparison

Tables 1, 2 illustrate the performance of contemporary classifiers for 40X, 100X, 200X and 400X magnification respectively. For each magnification, seven texture features out of which three are plain texture that directly extracts the feature from gray version of image, and other four are color texture that utilizes color-channel information are extracted.

From the tables following can be observed (for most or all cases):

(1) The performance when using color information (with or without stain normalization) is better performance than using gray level information. This highlights the importance of color in classification.

Table 1. Evaluation of color channel information along with contemporary classifiers for 40x and 100x. Best performance at each magnification is highlighted.

Image magnification			40x				100x			
Classifier and their variations			Linear SVM	Gaussian SVM	Gaussian KNN	Random forest	Linear SVM	Gaussian SVM	Gaussian KNN	Random forest
Plain texture features	GLCM	Gray scale	74.60	74.72	68.73	68.10	74.49	74.58	70.71	65.29
		Stain normalization	74.91	74.81	72.96	71.55	75.77	75.31	74.77	73.49
		Channel information	81.65	76.79	74.45	78.30	82.16	76.76	75.82	77.89
	CLBP	Gray scale	70.13	70.68	72.38	72.91	70.13	70.68	72.38	72.91
		Stain normalization	70.4	70.4	70.4	70.67	70.4	70.4	70.4	70.42
		Channel information	75.09	74.65	72.30	71.39	73.50	75.46	74.51	73.09
	LBQ	Gray scale	76.37	77.44	74.69	75.04	73.77	76.72	73.60	72.66
		Stain normalization	74.52	75.21	73.86	74.40	72.73	76.79	73.67	74.50
		Channel information	74.97	76.77	73.08	75.42	72.69	76.79	73.67	73.38
Colour texture feature	PFTAS	Gray scale	74.77	74.90	69.19	68.99	73.75	73.45	71.90	68.19
		Stain normalization	74.77	75.59	74.68	75.00	75.26	75.46	74.28	74.53
		Channel information	70.11	72.51	75.63	75.52	80.92	78.07	81.54	84.75
	Opponent LBP	Gray scale	73.86	70.22	71.62	72.36	75.42	74.58	74.62	70.55
		Stain normalization	76.09	75.25	75.54	76.05	68.66	75.88	74.27	71.92
		Channel information	**86.88**	86.20	85.41	85.18	86.17	86.40	85.09	87.41
	Gabour on gaussian color model	Gray scale	74.76	74.93	72.95	73.90	71.74	73.58	72.27	67.82
		Stain normalization	78.58	74.50	74.85	75.01	79.12	74.94	74.90	75.37
		Channel information	85.62	84.86	80.63	84.93	**88.41**	85.61	84.65	86.11
	M CCR (8)	Gray scale	73.83	70.4	67.80	68.06	69.74	70.4	68.76	65.63
		Stain normalization	72.35	74.40	72.78	71.18	71.83	73.25	70.87	75.67
		Channel information	78.93	78.50	82.63	84.42	80.40	78.96	80.30	87.15

Table 2. Evaluation of color channel information along with contemporary classifiers for 200x and 400x. Best performance at each magnification is highlighted.

Image magnification			200x				400x			
Classifier and their variations			Linear SVM	Gaussian SVM	Gaussian KNN	Random Forest	Linear SVM	Gaussian SVM	Gaussian KNN	Random Forest
Plain texture features	GLCM	Gray scale	70.37	71.10	69.73	63.80	70.06	69.57	70.46	66.03
		Stain normalization	71.98	72.67	70.18	68.88	69.28	70.08	72.33	70.51
		Channel information	84.19	81.24	76.98	82.61	78.45	77.21	74.30	76.14
	CLBP	Gray scale	62.85	68.93	66.65	63.31	65.69	69.46	68.56	63.68
		Stain normalization	70.4	70.4	70.4	70.67	70.42	70.29	62.08	69.89
		Channel information	73.48	71.19	73.52	70.29	72.96	72.54	72.85	70.26
	LBQ	Gray scale	72.86	75.34	74.27	72.08	72.93	74.99	73.73	70.55
		Stain normalization	73.76	75.50	74.48	71.94	75.97	75.48	74.28	72.52
		Channel information	73.94	75.24	74.04	73.16	75.59	75.33	73.92	69.79
Colour texture feature	PFTAS	Gray scale	71.71	70.56	70.91	65.13	72.22	71.92	70.10	64.00
		Stain normalization	74.17	73.08	73.89	72.73	75.54	74.79	75.19	72.30
		Channel information	73.52	75.46	74.51	72.80	77.14	74.31	77.18	80.97
	Opponent LBP	Gray scale	74.04	70.20	72.19	70.04	74.60	73.30	73.38	69.05
		Stain normalization	73.55	72.42	73.11	72.49	76.59	72.93	72.86	74.01
		Channel information	**88.86**	87.89	85.28	87.13	**87.55**	87.34	84.70	86.43
	Gabour on gaussian color model	Gray scale	65.28	67.29	67.17	61.10	71.67	69.48	68.86	67.70
		Stain normalization	79.56	74.43	73.16	75.11	77.55	73.59	72.92	75.93
		Channel information	87.76	88.19	85.49	85.75	85.66	86.83	83.93	82.62
	M CCR (8)	Gray scale	70.24	70.4	69.41	69.76	70.80	69.7	68.40	67.61
		Stain normalization	72.43	73.44	74.12	75.09	74.59	75.90	76.37	76.58
		Channel information	79.30	75.87	80.95	88.51	78.55	75.39	80.15	81.40

(2) Comparing the cases with and without stain normalization, it is seen that the classification performance is better in case of latter. However, the difference is not too high or even quite close in many cases where traditional texture features are used. This is expected as texture information is similar, except in some cases where even independent color channels may help in capturing the color variation.

(3) However, in case of joint color-texture features, except for a very few cases, the performance without stain normalization is consistently quite high. This indicates that the joint color-texture features, which consider the mutual dependency of color channels, indeed, better capture the color-texture variation for classification.

(4) It can also be observed that opponent LBP where opponent channels are considered to extract color channel information, shows the superior performance for most (three) of magnification images. However, Gabor feature on Gaussian color model, and M CCR also yield somewhat comparable performance.

There are very few exceptions from the above observations for some feature-classifier combinations. While these need to be better scrutinized, we note that most of the results support our hypothesis of the effectiveness of color-texture information in mitigating the need for stain normalization.

Finally, Table 4 compares the results of the proposed approach obtained with joint color-texture features, with some existing state-of art methods. In Table 4,

Table 3. Detailed description.   **Table 4.** Performance comparison.

	Magnifications				Total	Patient
	40x	100x	200x	400x		
Benign	625	644	623	588	2480	24
Malignant	1370	1437	1390	1232	5429	58
Total	1995	2081	2013	1820	7909	82

Methods & Score		[10]	[11]	[12]	Proposed
40x	Patient level	83.8 ± 4.1	90.6 ± 6.7	83.08 ± 2.08	86.88 ± 2.37
100x	Patient level	82.1 ± 4.9	88.4 ± 4.8	83.17 ± 3.51	**88.41 ± 2.73**
200x	Patient level	85.1 ± 3.1	84.6 ±	84.63 ± 2.72	**88.86 ± 3.76**
400x	Patient level	82.3 ± 3.8	86.1 ± 6.2	82.10 ± 4.42	**87.55 ± 3.01**

we report the best results of the proposed method obtained across various combination of color-texture descriptors and classifiers. We can observe that, except for the case of 40x, the proposed method outperforms the existing approaches. We also note from the Table 4 that at 400x, the obtained accuracy for most methods is lower than that at 100x and 200x. The reason could be that there are relatively less number of images for 400x and perhaps more data is required to capture the finer traits at higher magnification. Furthermore, one can also observe that the proposed work yields a lesser variance in scores, in most of the cases. This comparison further shows the effectiveness of joint color-texture features for classification.

4   Conclusion

In this work, we attempt to establish the usefulness of joint color-texture information, for classification without the need for stain normalization. We have experimented with various classifiers to show the importance of independent and dependent (mutual) color-channel information and find some interesting aspects about the same. From our experiments, it is apparent that joint dependency of color-texture can better capture the color-texture variability. We have also shown the role of contemporary classifiers with these sophisticated color-texture features. We believe that this is an interesting study which points towards obviating the need of stain normalization given effective features and classifiers. We also demonstrate that employing the joint color-texture features can also outperform the state-of-the-art methods for the breast cancer histopathology image classification.

References

1. Boyle, P., Levin, B., et al.: World cancer report 2008. IARC Press, International Agency for Research on Cancer (2008)
2. Bejnordi, B.E., Litjens, G., Timofeeva, N., Otte-Höller, I., Homeyer, A., Karssemeijer, N., van der Laak, J.A.W.M.: Stain specific standardization of whole-slide histopathological images. IEEE Trans. Med. Imaging **35**(2), 404–415 (2016)
3. Reinhard, E., Adhikhmin, M., Gooch, B., Shirley, P.: Color transfer between images. IEEE Comput. Graphics Appl. **21**(5), 34–41 (2001)
4. Vahadane, A., Peng, T., Sethi, A., Albarqouni, S., Wang, L., Baust, M., Steiger, K., Schlitter, A.M., Esposito, I., Navab, N.: Structure-preserving color normalization and sparse stain separation for histological images. IEEE Trans. Med. Imaging **35**(8), 1962–1971 (2016)

5. Basavanhally, A.N., Ganesan, S., Agner, S., Monaco, J.P., Feldman, M.D., Tomaszewski, J.E., Bhanot, G., Madabhushi, A.: Computerized image-based detection and grading of lymphocytic infiltration in her2+ breast cancer histopathology. IEEE Trans. Biomed. Eng. **57**(3), 642–653 (2010)
6. Ciompi, F., Geessink, O., Bejnordi, B.E., de Souza, G.S., Baidoshvili, A., Litjens, G., van Ginneken, B., Nagtegaal, I., van der Laak, J.: The importance of stain normalization in colorectal tissue classification with convolutional networks. arXiv preprint (2017). arXiv:1702.05931
7. Weingant, M., Reynolds, H.M., Haworth, A., Mitchell, C., Williams, S., DiFranco, M.D.: Ensemble prostate tumor classification in h&e whole slide imaging via stain normalization and cell density estimation. In: Zhou, L., Wang, L., Wang, Q., Shi, Y. (eds.) International Workshop on Machine Learning in Medical Imaging. LNCS, pp. 280–287. Springer, Cham (2015)
8. Fernández-Carrobles, M.M., Bueno, G., Déniz, O., Salido, J., García-Rojo, M., González-López, L.: Influence of texture and colour in breast TMA classification. PloS one **10**(10), e0141556 (2015)
9. Amaral, T., McKenna, S., Robertson, K., Thompson, A.: Classification of breast-tissue microarray spots using colour and local invariants. In: 5th IEEE International Symposium on Biomedical Imaging: From Nano to Macro, 2008. ISBI 2008, pp. 999–1002. IEEE (2008)
10. Spanhol, F.A., Oliveira, L.S., Petitjean, C., Heutte, L.: A dataset for breast cancer histopathological image classification. IEEE Trans. Biomed. Eng. **63**(7), 1455–1462 (2016)
11. Spanhol, F.A., Oliveira, L.S., Petitjean, C., Heutte, L.: Breast cancer histopathological image classification using convolutional neural networks. In: 2016 International Joint Conference on Neural Networks (IJCNN), pp. 2560–2567. IEEE (2016)
12. Bayramoglu, N., Kannala, J., Heikkilä, J.: Deep learning for magnification independent breast cancer histopathology image classification. In: 23rd International Conference on Pattern Recognition, ICPR 2016 (2016)
13. Krizhevsky, A., Sutskever, I., Hinton, G.E.: Imagenet classification with deep convolutional neural networks. In: Advances in neural information processing systems, pp. 1097–1105 (2012)
14. Haralick, R.M., Shanmugam, K., et al.: Textural features for image classification. IEEE Trans. Syst. Man Cybernet. **3**(6), 610–621 (1973)
15. Ojansivu, V., Heikkilä, J.: Blur insensitive texture classification using local phase quantization. In: Elmoataz, A., Lezoray, O., Nouboud, F., Mammass, D. (eds.) ICISP 2008. LNCS, vol. 5099, pp. 236–243. Springer, Heidelberg (2008). doi:10.1007/978-3-540-69905-7_27
16. Mäenpää, T., Pietikäinen, M.: Texture analysis with local binary patterns. Handbook Pattern Recog. Comput. Visi. **3**, 197–216 (2005)
17. Hoang, M.A., Geusebroek, J.-M., Smeulders, A.W.M.: Color texture measurement and segmentation. Sig. Process. **85**(2), 265–275 (2005)
18. Bianconi, F., Fernández, A., González, E., Caride, D., Calviño, A.: Rotation-invariant colour texture classification through multilayer CCR. Pattern Recogn. Lett. **30**(8), 765–773 (2009)
19. Hamilton, N.A., Pantelic, R.S., Hanson, K., Teasdale, R.D.: Fast automated cell phenotype image classification. BMC Bioinf. **8**(1), 110 (2007)
20. Classification-learner-app. https://in.mathworks.com/help/stats/classification-learner-app.html

Hybrid Tracking for Improved Registration of Laparoscopic Ultrasound and Laparoscopic Video for Augmented Reality

William Plishker[1]($\boxtimes$), Xinyang Liu[2], and Raj Shekhar[1,2]

[1] IGI Technologies, Inc., College Park, MD, USA
will@igitechnologies.com, RShekhar@childrensnational.org
[2] Sheikh Zayed Institute for Pediatric Surgical Innovation, Children's National Health System, Washington, DC, USA

Abstract. Laparoscopic *augmented reality* (AR), improves the surgeon's experience of using multimodal visual data during a procedure by fusion of medical image data (e.g., ultrasound images) onto live laparoscopic video. The majority of AR studies are based on either computer vision-based or hardware-based (e.g., optical and electromagnetic tracking) approaches. However, both approaches introduce registration errors because of variable operating conditions. To alleviate this problem, we propose a novel approach of hybrid tracking which comprises of both hardware-based and computer vision-based approaches. It consists of the registration of an ultrasound image with a time-matched video frame using electromagnetic tracking followed by a computer vision-based refinement of the registration and subsequent fusion. Experimental results demonstrate not only the feasibility of the proposed concept but also improved tracking accuracy that it provides and the potential for its integration into a future clinical AR system.

Keywords: Augmented reality · Laparoscopic ultrasound · Electromagnetic tracking · Hybrid tracking

1 Introduction

Laparoscopic surgery is an increasingly accepted mode of surgery because it is minimally invasive and leads to much faster recovery and improved outcomes. In a typical laparoscopic surgery, the primary means of intraoperative visualization is a real-time video of the surgical field acquired by a laparoscopic camera. Compared to open surgery, laparoscopic surgery lacks tactile feedback. Moreover, laparoscopic video is capable of providing only a surface view of the organs and cannot show anatomical structures beneath the exposed organ surfaces. One solution to this problem is augmented reality (AR), which is a method of overlaying imaging data—laparoscopic ultrasound (LUS) images in the present work—onto live laparoscopic video. Potential benefits of AR are improved procedure planning, improved surgical tool navigation and reduced procedure times. A typical AR approach consists of registration of real-time LUS images on live laparoscopic video followed by their superimposition.

© Springer International Publishing AG 2017
M.J. Cardoso et al. (Eds.): CARE/CLIP 2017, LNCS 10550, pp. 170–179, 2017.
DOI: 10.1007/978-3-319-67543-5_17

Image-to-video registration methods can be divided into two broad categories: (1) computer vision (CV)-based and (2) hardware-based methods. The first category uses CV techniques to track in real time natural anatomical landmarks and/or user-introduced patterns within the field of view of the camera used. When ultrasound is the augmenting imaging modality, tracking the ultrasound transducer in the video is the goal in these approaches. For example, some earlier methods [1, 2] attached user-defined patterns on the ultrasound transducer and tracked those patterns in the video. Feuerstein et al. [3], on the other hand, directly tracked the LUS transducer in the video by detecting lines describing the outer contours of the probe. However, the CV-based approaches may fail or degrade in the presence of occlusion and variable lighting conditions [4].

The second category concerns the use of external tracking hardware devices. The most established method at present is optical tracking, which uses infrared cameras to track optical markers affixed rigidly on the desired tools and imaging devices. The method has been employed in many AR applications [5–7]. AR systems based on electromagnetic (EM) tracking have also been proposed [8, 9]. Tracking hardware is susceptible to two types of errors: system and calibration. The system-based errors in EM tracking often stem from ferrous metals and conductive materials in tools that are close enough to the field generator [10]. Optical markers frequently face the line-of-sight problem. Calibration-based registration errors could be associated with experimental errors from system calibration, which includes ultrasound calibration [11] and laparoscopic camera calibration [12].

We propose a novel hybrid tracking method comprising of both hardware-based and vision-based methods, which may provide consistent, more accurate and reliable image fusion for an AR system. In this work, we focus on applying our method to EM tracking that is capable of tracking the LUS transducer with a flexible imaging tip. The same framework can also be applied to optical tracking. After an ultrasound image is registered with and overlaid on a time-matched video frame using EM tracking, a vision-based algorithm is used to refine the registration and subsequent fusion. Such a rectified calibration method can be accomplished in two stages by: (1) computing a correction transformation which when applied to a 3D Computer Aided Design (CAD) model of the LUS probe improves the alignment of its projection with the actual LUS probe visible in the camera image and (2) incorporating the calculated correction transformation in the overall calibration system.

2 Methods

Our AR system in this study includes a clinical vision system (Image 1 Hub, KARL STORZ, Tuttlingen, Germany) with a 10-mm 0° laparoscopic camera (Image 1 HD), an ultrasound scanner (Flex Focus 700, BK Ultrasound, Analogic Corporation, Peabody, MA, USA) with a 9-mm LUS transducer with a flexible imaging tip (Model 8836-RF), an EM tracking system with a tabletop field generator (Aurora, Northern Digital Inc., Waterloo, ON, Canada), and a graphics processing unit (GPU)-accelerated laptop computer that runs the image fusion software. As shown in Fig. 1, we designed and 3D-printed a wedge-like mount to hold the EM sensor (Aurora 6DOF Flex Tube, Type 2, 1.3 mm diameter) using an existing biopsy needle introducer track in the LUS transducer [9]. The mount was made as thin as possible so that the integrated transducer can still go through a 12-mm trocar, a typical-sized trocar for use with the original transducer.

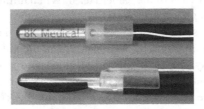

Fig. 1. Custom-designed EM tracking mount on the LUS transducer.

The outline of our hybrid tracking framework is illustrated in Fig. 2. It has two main stages. The first stage consists of two parts: (1) computing calibration of AR system components: laparoscope and LUS transducer; (2) registration of LUS image and the projection of the 3D LUS transducer model on the camera image using the calibration results. In the second stage, the 2D projection of the 3D LUS transducer model is fitted to the actual transducer seen in the camera image. To achieve this, the position and pose parameters of the 3D LUS transducer model are optimized to determine the best fit of its projection to the camera image. Such a correction transformation matrix is fed back to Stage 1, and thus the registration of the LUS image to video is refined.

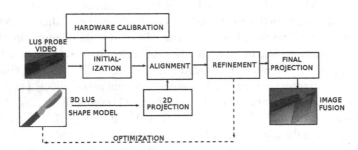

Fig. 2. The outline of the proposed framework.

2.1 System Calibration for AR

We first briefly describe the method for our hardware-based AR visualization. Let $p_{US} = [x\,y\,0\,1]^T$ denote a point in the LUS image in homogeneous coordinates, in which the z coordinate is 0. Let $p_{Lap}^U = [u\,v\,1]^T$ denote the point that p_{US} corresponds to in the undistorted camera image. If we denote T_A^B as the 4×4 transformation matrix from the coordinate system of A to that of B, the registration of p_{US} on the undistorted camera image can be expressed as

$$p_{Lap}^U = C \cdot [I_3 0] \cdot T_{Mark\text{-}Lap}^{Cam} \cdot T_{Tracker}^{Mark\text{-}Lap} \cdot T_{Mark\text{-}US}^{Tracker} \cdot T_{US}^{Mark\text{-}US} \cdot p_{US} \qquad (1)$$

where US refers to the LUS image; Mark-US refers to the EM sensor attached on the LUS transducer; Tracker refers to the EM tracker; Mark-Lap refers to the EM sensor attached on the laparoscope; Cam refers to the laparoscopic camera; I_3 is an identity matrix of size 3; and C is the camera matrix. $T^{\text{Mark-US}}_{\text{US}}$ can be obtained from ultrasound calibration; $T^{\text{Tracker}}_{\text{Mark-US}}$ and $T^{\text{Mark-Lap}}_{\text{Tracker}}$ can be obtained from tracking system; $T^{\text{Cam}}_{\text{Mark-Lap}}$ and C can be obtained from laparoscope calibration [12].

2.2 Improved System Calibration for AR

To refine the registration of the LUS image, we first project a 3D LUS transducer model on the camera image using the standard calibration results. We then apply a vision-based algorithm to register the projected 3D transducer model with the actual LUS transducer shown in the video. This yields a correction matrix T_{Corr} as a rigid transformation. Since there is a fixed geometric relationship between the LUS transducer and the LUS image, the same T_{Corr} can be used to refine the location of the LUS image overlaid on the video. As an update to Eq. 1, a summary of our general approach can be expressed as

$$p^{\text{U}}_{\text{Lap}} = C \cdot [I_3 0] \cdot T_{\text{Corr}} \cdot T^{\text{Cam}}_{\text{Mark-Lap}} \cdot T^{\text{Mark-Lap}}_{\text{Tracker}} \cdot T^{\text{Tracker}}_{\text{Mark-US}} \cdot T^{\text{Mark-US}}_{\text{US}} \cdot T^{\text{US}}_{\text{Model}} \cdot P_{\text{Model}} \qquad (2)$$

where points of the 3D LUS transducer model are first transferred to the LUS image coordinate system through $T^{\text{US}}_{\text{Model}}$, which is described in the next section.

2.3 LUS Probe Model and Calibrations

We obtained a CAD model of the LUS probe used in this study from the manufacturer. Because the exact mechanical relationship between the imaging tip of the LUS transducer and the LUS image is proprietary information and not known to the research community, we developed a simple registration step to transfer the coordinate system of the CAD model to that of the LUS image (supposing the LUS image space is 3D with $z = 0$). As illustrated in Fig. 3, we selected three characteristic points on the CAD model and their corresponding points on the LUS image plane. Without loss of generality, we fixed the scan depth of the LUS image to 6.4 cm, a commonly used depth setting for ultrasound imaging during abdominal procedures. A simple three-point rigid registration was then performed to obtain $T^{\text{US}}_{\text{Model}}$ in Eq. 2.

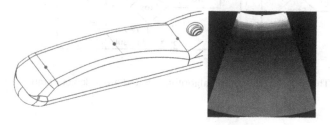

Fig. 3. The three points selected on the LUS CAD model (left) and on the LUS image (right).

We performed ultrasound calibration using the tools provided in the PLUS library [11]. Laparoscope calibration was performed using the fast approach of [12], which requires only a single image of the calibration pattern.

2.4   Model Projection and Alignment

To compare the pose and position of the rendered virtual model and the probe in the camera image, we propose the workflow of the CV-based refinement algorithm as presented in Fig. 4. First a region of interest (ROI) is generated for each frame of the laparoscopic video using fast visual tracking based on robust discriminative correlation filters [13] such that subsequent processing focuses on the imaging tip. Based on this coarse estimate of the probe's location, the bounding box surrounding the imaging tip is intended to include at least some portion of the top, middle, and tip of the probe as seen by the camera. To find the straight edges of these features of the probe, the camera image is first converted to a gray scale image based on brightness, followed by Canny edge detection. We used the Probabilistic Hough Transform (PHT) to extract a set of lines from the edge detection result within the ROI, an example of which is shown in Fig. 5. The line set was filtered by creating a coarse grain 2D histogram with the axes defined by PHT parameters (r, θ) and values of histogram defined by the sum of the lengths of lines in the bin. All lines not contained within the highest peak present in the 2D histogram are removed to produce a set of lines that corresponds with the long edges, parallel or close to parallel present in the probe. From this smaller set of lines, a fine grain 2D histogram based on the PHT parameters (r, θ) is created. The two highest peaks in this histogram represent the top and middle of the probe. The indices of the peaks are then used in the cost function for the optimization of the virtual probe location.

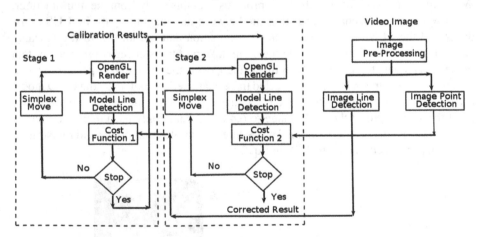

Fig. 4. The proposed refinement algorithm. Dotted areas depict iterative processes.

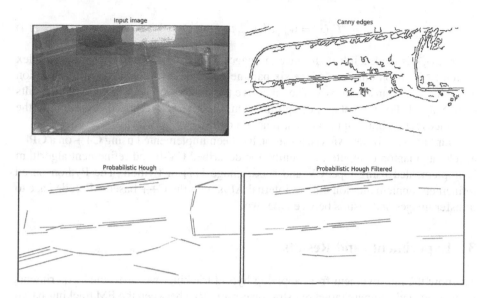

Fig. 5. An example of the hybrid based tracking system with intermediate results displayed: Top Left – gray scale representation of the original camera image and the mask box being used shown in red, Top Right – Canny edges detected within the mask, Lower Left – Probabilistic Hough Transform line set from Canny, Lower Right – line feature based filtering of the line set (Color figure online)

In Stage 1 of optimization, we use the same procedure to detect the same two feature lines both for the rendered 3D LUS transducer model and for the actual transducer shown in the camera image. We compared the alignment of the feature lines using a cost function defined as

$$F_1(x) = \sum\nolimits_{i=1}^{2} \left[w_r \cdot \left(r_{\text{img}}^i - r_{\text{gl}}^i(x) \right)^2 + w_\theta \cdot \left(\theta_{\text{img}}^i - \theta_{\text{gl}}^i(x) \right)^2 \right] \tag{3}$$

where w is a scalar, *img* refers to the camera image, and *gl* refers to the OpenGL-rendered 3D LUS transducer model. The optimization used the simplex method [15] to search for the five parameters x associated with a rigid transformation (T_{Corr} in Eq. 2). In our current work, we fixed the other parameter, i.e., the one associated with the rotation about the LUS transducer axis. With only two feature lines as constraints, the optimization in Stage 1 may not accurately estimate parameters associated with translation along the LUS transducer axis.

In Stage 2 of optimization, we detect a feature point of the tip of the probe in both images to address inaccuracies along the transducer axis. We used gradient descent-based active contours method [14] to segment the LUS probe from the camera image and identify a feature point p as the farthest point corresponding with the tip of the transducer. The initialization for segmentation was provided by an ellipse encompassing the ROI. We compared the feature points using another cost function

$$F_2(x) = w_p \cdot d\left(p_{\text{img}}, p_{\text{gl}}(x)\right)^2 \tag{4}$$

where $d(\cdot, \cdot)$ is the Euclidean distance in image. In this stage, we restricted the simplex search to focus on only one of the six parameters: the one associated with translation along the LUS transducer axis. The other five parameters are kept fixed to their results from Stage 1. For both stages of optimization, the search terminated according to the tolerances set on both input and cost function deltas.

Our hardware-based AR visualization has been implemented using C++ on a GPU-accelerated laptop computer. Currently, the described CV-based refinement algorithm is implemented using OpenCV and scikit-image [17] in Python. The Python based refinement implementation utilizes internal APIs with the C++ based AR code base to transfer images and results between the two.

3   Experiments and Results

To show the improvement from applying hybrid tracking, we performed experiments to measure and compare target registration error (TRE) between the EM tracking-based approach and the hybrid approach. A target point, the intersection of two cross wires immersed in a water tank, was imaged using the LUS transducer. The target point along with the imaging tip of the LUS transducer was viewed with the laparoscope, whose lens was immersed in water as well. The LUS image was overlaid on the camera image through the EM tracking-based approach (Sect. 2.1) as well as the hybrid approach. The target point in the overlaid LUS image can then be identified and compared with the actual target point shown in the camera image. Their Euclidean distance in the image plane is the TRE.

We performed experiments with four different poses of the laparoscope and the LUS transducer. The average TRE of the EM tracking-based approach was measured to be 102.0 ± 60.5 pixel (8.2 ± 4.9 mm), and that of the hybrid approach was 46.7 ± 10.1 pixel (3.8 ± 0.8 mm) with an image resolution of the camera of 1920×1280. The hybrid approach improved overlay accuracy of the original EM tracking-based approach. The CV-based refinement process took on average 52 s, the major bottleneck being the C++ API interface required to read in a new candidate correction matrix. The total number of iteration steps in optimization was fewer than 110 steps for examples tried. Figure 6 shows an example of the refinement results.

We also tested our approach with a more realistic camera and ultrasound images by testing images from phantom. While we did not have a quantitative evaluation of such images, we confirmed that the image processing and subsequent optimization qualitatively worked as well as in the wire phantom. Figure 7 shows examples of this evaluation.

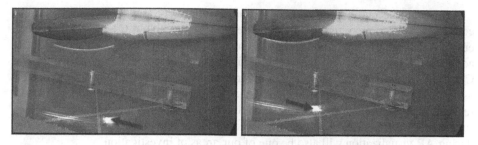

Fig. 6. Example of vision-based refinement showing the initial AR visualization using the EM tracking approach (left), and corrected AR visualization using the hybrid tracking approach (right). The arrow indicates the target point shown in the overlaid LUS image.

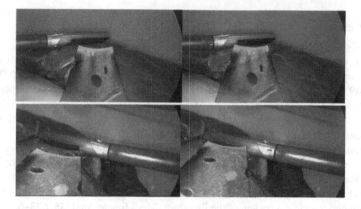

Fig. 7. Two examples of vision-based refinement on an abdominal phantom. The initial AR visualization (left) and corrected AR visualization using the hybrid tracking approach (right).

4   Discussion and Conclusion

In this work, we developed a computer vision-based refinement method to correct registration error in hardware-based AR visualization. Initial hardware-based registration is essential to our approach because it provides an ROI for robust feature line detection, as well as a relatively close initialization for simplex-based optimization. We have developed a vision-based solution to refine image-to-video registration obtained using hardware-based tracking. A 3D LUS transducer model was first projected on the camera image based on calibration results and tracking data. The model was then registered with the actual LUS transducer using image processing and simplex optimization. Finally, the resulting correction matrix was applied to the ultrasound image. The method is promising as evidenced by our preliminary results included in this work. After further refinement, the proposed hybrid framework could greatly improve the accuracy and robustness of a laparoscopic AR system for clinical use.

Although the current computational time is relatively lengthy even for periodic correction, we can more tightly integrate the algorithm with our C++ and GPU-accelerated AR system in the future. If implemented on GPU, the Hough Transform can be achieved in 3 ms [16], and the entire refinement process could take less than 1 s. Currently, Stage 1 of the optimization algorithm only used five of the six parameters associated with a rigid transformation. The rotation about the LUS probe axis is not refined. In the future, we will include the refinement of this parameter in our algorithm. In addition, determining how often the vision-based refinement should be repeated during AR visualization will also be one of our areas of investigation.

Acknowledgement. This work was supported by the National Institutes of Health/National Cancer Institute under Grant CA192504.

References

1. Leven, J., et al.: DaVinci canvas: a telerobotic surgical system with integrated, robot-assisted, laparoscopic ultrasound capability. In: Duncan, J.S., Gerig, G. (eds.) MICCAI 2005. LNCS, vol. 3749, pp. 811–818. Springer, Heidelberg (2005). doi:10.1007/11566465_100
2. Pratt, P., Jaeger, A., Hughes-Hallett, A., Mayer, E., Vale, J., Darzi, A., Peters, T., Yang, G.Z.: Robust ultrasound probe tracking: initial clinical experiences during robot-assisted partial nephrectomy. Int. J. Comput. Assist. Radiol. Surg. 10(12), 1905–1913 (2015)
3. Feuerstein, M., Reichl, T., Vogel, J., Traub, J., Navab, N.: New approaches to online estimation of electromagnetic tracking errors for laparoscopic ultrasonography. Comput. Aided Surg. 13(5), 311–323 (2008)
4. Bouget, D., Allan, M., Stoyanov, D., Jannin, P.: Vision-based and marker-less surgical tool detection and tracking: a review of the literature. Med. Image Anal. 35, 633–654 (2017)
5. Feuerstein, M., Mussack, T., Heining, S.M., Navab, N.: Intraoperative laparoscope augmentation for port placement and resection planning in minimally invasive liver resection. IEEE Trans. Med. Imaging 27(3), 355–369 (2008)
6. Shekhar, R., Dandekar, O., Bhat, V., Philip, M., Lei, P., Godinez, C., Sutton, E., George, I., Kavic, S., Mezrich, R., Park, A.: Live augmented reality: a new visualization method for laparoscopic surgery using continuous volumetric computed tomography Surg. Endosc. 24(8), 1976–1985 (2010)
7. Kang, X., Azizian, M., Wilson, E., Wu, K., Martin, A.D., Kane, T.D., Peters, C.A., Cleary, K., Shekhar, R.: Stereoscopic augmented reality for laparoscopic surgery. Surg. Endosc. 28(7), 2227–2235 (2014)
8. Cheung, C.L., Wedlake, C., Moore, J., Pautler, S.E., Peters, T.M.: Fused video and ultrasound images for minimally invasive partial nephrectomy: a phantom study. In: Jiang, T., Navab, N., Pluim, J.P.W., Viergever, M.A. (eds.) MICCAI 2010. LNCS, vol. 6363, pp. 408–415. Springer, Heidelberg (2010). doi:10.1007/978-3-642-15711-0_51
9. Liu, X., Kang, S., Plishker, W., Zaki, G., Kane, T.D., Shekhar, R.: Laparoscopic stereoscopic augmented reality: toward a clinically viable electromagnetic tracking solution. J. Med. Imaging (Bellingham) 3(4), 045001 (2016)
10. Franz, A.M., Haidegger, T., Birkfellner, W., Cleary, K., Peters, T.M., Maier-Hein, L.: Electromagnetic tracking in medicine – a review of technology, validation, and applications. IEEE Trans. Med. Imaging 33(8), 1702–1725 (2014)

11. Lasso, A., Heffter, T., Rankin, A., Pinter, C., Ungi, T., Fichtinger, G.: PLUS: open-source toolkit for ultrasound-guided intervention systems. IEEE Trans. Biomed. Eng. **61**(10), 2527–2537 (2014)
12. Liu, X., Plishker, W., Zaki, G., Kang, S., Kane, T.D., Shekhar, R.: On-demand calibration and evaluation for electromagnetically tracked laparoscope in augmented reality visualization. Int. J. Comput. Assist. Radiol. Surg. **11**(6), 1163–1171 (2016)
13. Danelljan, M., Häger, G., Khan, F., Felsberg, M.: Accurate Scale Estimation for Robust Visual Tracking. BMCV (2014)
14. Chan, T.F., Vese, L.A.: Active contours without edges. IEEE Trans. Image Process. **10**(2), 266–277 (2001)
15. Nelder, J.A., Mead, R.A.: A simplex method for function minimization. Comput. J. **7**, 308–313 (1965)
16. van den Braak, G.-J., Nugteren, C., Mesman, B., Corporaal, H.: Fast Hough Transform on GPUs: exploration of algorithm trade-offs. In: Blanc-Talon, J., Kleihorst, R., Philips, W., Popescu, D., Scheunders, P. (eds.) ACIVS 2011. LNCS, vol. 6915, pp. 611–622. Springer, Heidelberg (2011). doi:10.1007/978-3-642-23687-7_55
17. van der Walt, S., Schönberger, J., Nunez-Iglesias, J., Boulogne, F., Warner, J., Yager, N., Gouillart, E., Yu, T., The scikit-image Contributors: scikit-image scikit-image: Image processing in Python. PeerJ **2**, e453 (2014). http://dx.doi.org/10.7717/peerj.453

Author Index

Abugharbieh, Rafeef   124
Alvarez, Jose   50
Angermann, Quentin   29
Armin, Mohammad Ali   50

Baba, Masahi   16
Barnes, Nick   50
Bernal, Jorge   29
Bhavsar, Arnav   160
Braxton, Vaughn   99

Cooper, Anthony   124
Cootes, Tim   91
Cuadra, Meritxell Bach   141
Cygert, Sebastian   3

Daisne, Jean-François   133
de Frutos, Noelia Cubero   151
De, Smita   99
Diez-Ferrer, Marta   151
Dray, Xavier   29

Ebsim, Raja   91
Enquobahrie, Andinet   116
Ensel, Scott   116

Fernández-Esparrach, Gloria   29
Furukawa, Ryo   16

Gil, Debora   151
Grimpen, Florian   50
Gupta, Vibha   160

Hacihaliloglu, Ilker   108
Hammami, Maroua   29
Hayashi, Yuichiro   60
Herrell, S. Duke   99
Histace, Aymeric   29
Hiura, Shinsaku   16
Hodgson, Antony J.   124

Hu, Qingmao   42
Huo, Yuankai   99

Jia, Fucang   42
Jorge, João   141
Jung, Florian   133

Kawasaki, Hiroshi   16
Keating, Robert   116

Landman, Bennett   99
Leibetseder, Andreas   70
Levivier, Marc   141
Li, Hongdong   50
Linguraru, Marius George   116
Liu, Xinyang   170
Luo, Huoling   42

Maeder, Philippe   141
Marques, José P.   141
Medea, Biebl-Rydlo   133
Minchole, Elisa   151
Misawa, Kazunari   60
Miyazaki, Daisuke   16
Mori, Kensaku   60
Mulpuri, Kishore   124
Mwikirize, Cosmas   108

Naito, Masahito   16
Najdenovska, Elena   141
Naqvi, Jawad   91
Nosher, John L.   108

Oda, Masahiro   60
Oh, Albert   116
Ortiz, Rosa Maria   151

Paniagua, Beatriz   116
Paserin, Olivia   124
Petscharnig, Stefan   70
Plishker, William   170

Porras, Antonio R.   116
Primus, Manfred Jürgen   70

Ramos-Terrades, Oriol   151
Rogers, Gary F.   116
Romain, Olivier   29
Rosell, Antoni   151
Roth, Holger   60

Salvado, Olivier   50
Sanchez, Carles   151
Sánchez, F. Javier   29
Sánchez-Montes, Cristina   29
Sanomura, Yoji   16
Schoeffmann, Klaus   70
Shao, Jinliang   42

Sharma, Kartikeya   160
Shekhar, Raj   170
Singh, Apurva   160

Tanaka, Shinji   16
Thiran, Jean-Philippe   141
Tsering, Deki   116
Tu, Liyun   116
Tuleasca, Constantin   141

Wang, Cheng   60
Wesarg, Stefan   133
Wesierski, Daniel   3

Xiao, Deqiang   42

Printed in the United States
By Bookmasters